The Ki Process

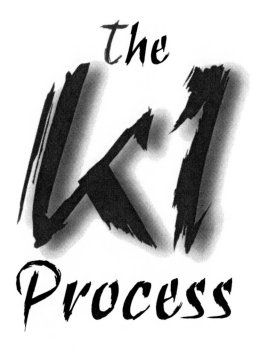

the Ki Process

Korean Secrets for Cultivating Dynamic Energy

SCOTT SHAW

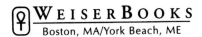

WEISERBOOKS
Boston, MA/York Beach, ME

First published in 1997 by
Red Wheel/Weiser, LLC
York Beach, ME
With offices at
368 Congress Street
Boston, MA 02210
www.redwheelweiser.com

Library of Congress Cataloging-in-Publication Data

Shaw, Scott
      The ki process: Korean secrets for cultivating dynamic energy /
Scott Shaw
        p.   cm.
      Includes index.
      ISBN 0-87728-879-8 (paper : alk. paper)
      1. Ch'i (Chinese philosophy)   2. Mind and body—Korea.
      I. Title.
      BF127.C49S48   1997
      181'.119--dc21   96-39551
                                           CIP

MG
Typeset in 10.5 Berkeley Book
Cover and text design by Kathryn Sky-Peck
Cover painting copyright © 1997 Hae Won Shin

Printed in the United States of America

08 07 06 05
10 9 8 7 6 5 4

TABLE OF CONTENTS

Part I

Introduction to the Ki Concept

Part II

The Meridians: Passageways of ki

Part III
The Mastery of ki

LIST OF ILLUSTRATIONS

LIST OF TABLES

ACKNOWLEDGMENT

Special thanks to Joan D. Albert, Ph.D., for her enlightened support throughout the creation of this book.

NOTE TO THE READER

The information provided in this book is not intended to replace the service of a physician. The material is presented for educational purposes and for self-help. The author and the publishers are in no way responsible for any medical claims regarding the material presented.

INTRODUCTION

*T*hrough modern science we learn that every element of this universe we inhabit is in motion, from the smallest subatomic particle to the largest planet. This motion is fueled by a constant, unceasing energy. Science has no defined name for it. In Asia, since ancient times, this energy has been known as Ki.

Ki is a universal energy. It flows through all things. Since Ki is present in all things, we, as participants in this energy, have the ability to tap into it consciously, through prescribed methods.

Ki is not the energy of an individual person; that is, personal strength. Ki can, however, be isolated and put to use by an individual.

Ki is not like a muscle which, through physical exercise, can be developed and strengthened. Development of your ability to utilize Ki comes through refining your mental clarity and your understanding of the way this universal energy intermingles with your body.

Ki cannot be harnessed. There is no savings account in the human body for Ki. Though Ki cannot be captured, it can be consciously received, focalized, and isolated, thereby bringing it into the realm of personal usage when the physical or mental need arises. From the science of thermodynamics, we learn that no energy in this universe can be created or destroyed; it can only be moved from one location to the next. This modern confirmation of ancient Ki understanding, confirms what the practitioners of Ki have proven for hundreds of generations: that we can focalize and harness great amounts of energy, both physical and mental, and then use this energy to achieve current needs.

The undisciplined use of Ki can be illustrated ideally by the people who remarkably lift away a several-hundred pound boulder which has fallen on a loved one. Some way, somehow, these average individuals are able to harness superhuman power and save a person's life. Through the practice of defined Ki developmental exercises, you, too, can learn how to harness this energy, which is in abundant supply throughout the universe, and channel it into yourself to be used in times of need.

The development and understanding of Ki is not only a way to tap into superior physical power; it is a method to focus mental strength as well. By focalizing Ki through the techniques discussed in this book, you will have a much clearer perception of the world around you—and how to substantially pinpoint your mental energies to achieve whatever mental task is at hand.

Ki was first described in the *Huang Ti Nei Ching Su Wen* (*The Yellow Emperor's Classic of Internal Medicine*). This text was created in China in the third century B.C. and was the first written document to describe how Ki energy enters, flows through, and then exits the human body. From China, this knowledge was passed on to the Korean peninsula in approximately 200 B.C. Once the principles of Ki had been absorbed into the Korean understanding of body and mind, the Hwa Rang (Flowering Youth) warriors of the Korean peninsula were the first to redefine Ki and use it as a way to enhance physical and mental power, thus making the science of Ki uniquely Korean.

Over the past several centuries, the practice of Ki has been utilized predominantly by acupuncturists, acupressurists, and martial artists. This does not mean, however, that the average person cannot utilize it as well. Modern society often times leaves the average individual in tremendous need of additional physical and mental energy. These early practitioners of Ki simply laid the groundwork for their ancient knowledge to be spread to the masses.

Ki is not an abstract science accessible only to holy men. It is a defined science that you, as an average individual, can put into use in your daily life from the first moment you begin to practice the very basic Ki-developing exercises. In the pages that follow, I will discuss how Ki was understood and used from ancient Korea to modern times, and how you can put this science to use in everyday life to acquire better health and more physical and mental energy.

Part I

☯

Introduction to the Ki Concept

THE HISTORICAL FOUNDATIONS OF KI

*I*n order to begin your work with Ki energy, you must first possess a basic understanding of Asian medicine. This knowledge will greatly enhance your path to Ki mastery. While most people who read this book may already possess a knowledge of the terms which relate to Ki science, a brief overview follows for those of you who may not be familiar with the terminology. Even if you are familiar with this work, this section will introduce you to the terms I will be using in subsequent sections.

THE NEI CHING

The *Huang Ti Nei Ching Su Wen* (*The Yellow Emperor's Classic of Internal Medicine*), commonly referred to as the *Nei Ching*, was the first written text ever to discuss Ki (internal energy) and its interrelationship with the human body. In the *Nei Ching*, Ki is described as the "universal energy" which nourishes and sustains all life.

The *Nei Ching* is written in the form of a dialogue on the subject of healing between the Yellow Emperor, Huang-ti, and his minister, Chi-po. Huang-ti was a mythological ruler of China, whom legend claims to have lived from 2697 to 2599 B.C. He is said to have invented most aspects of Chinese culture. Though Chinese folklore claims the *Nei Ching* was written during the life of Huang-ti, historians date the book at approximately 300 B.C., during the Warring States period of Chinese history.

The *Nei Ching* not only describes Ki, but extensively details the functions of the human body. It represents an incredible accomplishment for this text to have been conceived and written by metaphysicians and medical practitioners of this time period, for along with a relatively correct detailed internal anatomy of the human body, the *Nei Ching* was the first text ever to detail blood circulation. The concept of blood circulation and its effect on the human body was described in the *Nei Ching* 2,000 years before European medical science "discovered" it in the 16th century.

The *Nei Ching* describes how Ki circulation in the human body is directed by invisible circulation channels known as meridians. The meridians are named for the major body organ or the bodily function they impact: i.e., the Heart Meridian, the Lung Meridian, the Conceptual Meridian, and so on. Located along these meridians are precise access points which allow the trained individual to stimulate the flow of Ki, thus nourishing and healing the body with accelerated Ki current.

The *Nei Ching* claims that if an individual is ill, listless, or having any physical or mental problems, the Ki flow along one or more meridian is blocked. This Ki-flow blockage can be due to the body's Yin and Yang being out of balance. To remedy this imbalance and restore proper Ki circulation, Chinese physicians of this time period developed acupuncture to stimulate the flow of Ki in the human body. This medical practice and those it spawned are still in use today.

YIN (UM) AND YANG

The concept of Yin (*Um* in Korean) and Yang is no doubt the theory most integral to understanding not only Ki energy but the Asian mindset toward life and the universe as a whole. This fundamental concept of universal duality extends at least as far back as the eighth century B.C. in China.

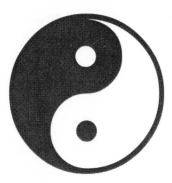

Figure 1. The Yin/Yang symbol.

The Yin and Yang philosophy was developed by thinkers who watched all aspects of the functioning world which surrounded them. They came to the conclusion that all life exists as a duality. For example, there can be no day without night. There can be no hot without cold. There can be no life without death. With this theory as a central focus, Chinese philosophers concluded that everything is in a constant state of flux attempting to find a balance between these two polar dualities.

In Yin and Yang philosophy, Yin is the negative and Yang is the positive. Yin is the earth; Yang is the heavens. Yin is cold; Yang is hot. Yin is female; Yang is male. Yin is emptiness; Yang is fullness. Yin is white; Yang is black.

In the symbol which came to represent Yin and Yang, there appears a white dot on a black field and a black dot on a white field (see figure 1). This demonstrates that within all Yang there is the essence of Yin, and within all that is Yin, there is a trace of Yang. Throughout the continuous evolution of the world, these opposites have given birth to one another.

In the *Nei Ching*, health is seen as a harmony between the Yin and Yang forces and illness is an imbalance of the two. Yin and Yang are equal powers but are in constant motion, causing continual change. To remain healthy, one must constantly redefine the balance between the two. The primary role of the physician is to restore the balance between the Yin and Yang in an ailing individual.

For the practitioner of Ki, Yin and Yang comprise duality which one must experience and with which one must come into harmony by understanding the particular defining aspects of each element. In this way, Ki energy may be utilized and directed in a fashion which is acceptable by nature. Thus no imbalances between the two energies will be created.

THE FIVE ELEMENTS

In association with the dualitistic concept of Yin and Yang, Chinese philosophers and physicians, witnessing the process of continual change in the world around them, organized these changes into five specific categories known as the Five Earthly Elements. These five elements are: fire (*Pul*), earth (*Chi-gu*), metal (*Kum-sok*), water (*Mul*), and wood (*Na-mu*). Each of these elements has its own individual attributes which affect not only the health and well-being of the human body, but the state of the world as well. (See Tables 1 and 2, pages 6 and 7).

As stated in the *Nei Ching*, all of the five elements are continually present within the human body. The amount and balance of each element is in proportion to the other elements and is dominated by Yin or by Yang.

Table 1. The Attributes of the Five Elements.

Fire:	Hot, dry, destructive, moving	Water:	Cool, wet, flowing, yielding
Earth:	Constant, life-giving, fertile	Wood:	Rooted, growing, living
Metal:	Hard, firm, conductive		

Table 2. The Five Elements and their Physical Associations.

	FIRE	EARTH	METAL	WATER	WOOD
Season	Summer	Late Summer	Autumn	Winter	Spring
Climate	Hot	Rainy	Dry	Cold	Windy
Direction	South	Home	West	North	East
Emotion	Happiness	Reflective	Unhappy	Fear	Anger
Color	Yellow	Blue	White	Black	Red
Yin Organ	Heart	Spleen	Lungs	Kidney	Liver
Yang Organ	Small Intestine	Stomach	Large Intestine	Bladder	Gall Bladder

Each element exists within its own time cycle of Creation, Interaction, and, finally, Destruction. The time cycles of the five elements are defined by Earth's interrelationship with the Sun, and thus relate to the time of day.

As time moves forward, each of the five elements flows into its own Cycle of Creation. As it does, it destroys the previous element. Thus, the fire element creates the earth element. During the transitional period of time between Earth Element Creation and Fire Element Destruction, they are interactive. Both of their individual characteristics are prevalent in the world as each individual element continues on its path of nonceasing creation, interaction, and destruction (see figure 2, page 8).

Each meridian of the human body is activated by one of these five elements (see Table 3, page 9). Each meridian is additionally dominated by Yin or Yang. As each of the five elements has a specified time period when it is most active, the human body is directly affected by the duration of the element's presence. Therefore, the flow of Ki into the body and how one utilizes Ki is directly related to the interaction of the five elements.

From ancient China, through ancient Korea, and even today, a homeopathic doctor will diagnose either an overabundance or a deficiency of one or more of the five elements in the body of a patient who is ill, unhappy, or disassociated from the world. To effect a cure, herbal medicines, acupuncture, acupressure, or dietary changes are prescribed to rebalance the five elements in the body, thus realigning Yin and Yang.

To the modern mind, it is somewhat difficult to conceive that an earthly element such as fire, earth, metal, water, or wood has anything to

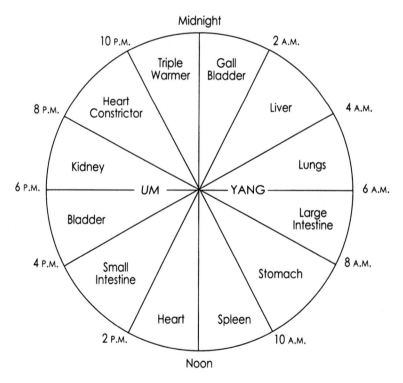

Figure 2. Meridian timetable.

Table 3. Yin (*Um*) and Yang.

ELEMENT	YIN (UM)	YANG
Fire Element	Heart Meridian	Small Intestine Meridian
Earth Element	Spleen Meridian	Stomach Meridian
Metal Element	Lung Meridian	Large Intestine Meridian
Water Element	Kidney Meridian	Bladder Meridian
Wood Element	Liver Meridian	Gall Bladder Meridian

do with the overall balance or health of the individual. It must be remembered that these five elements are not actual physical entities in the body. They are, however, descriptions of specific states which exist within the human body and mind. If an overabundance or a deficiency of any of these states exists, it can cause a susceptibility to ill health. To this end, what the five elements represent in today's world is a method of gauging the overall physical and mental makeup of a specific person. Once the physician has gauged this, balancing methods may be put into action to make any person more healthy and emotionally whole.

THE EXPANSION OF KI KNOWLEDGE THROUGHOUT ANCIENT ASIA

From the third century B.C., the *Nei Ching* set the standards for Chinese medicine and the defined knowledge of Ki. This knowledge was passed on predominantly by monks and priests who were the healers of ancient Asia. From China, the knowledge of Ki traveled first to Korea and then, much later, from Korea to Japan.

• Ancient Korea •

Formalized Chinese contact with the Korean peninsula began in approximately 200 B.C., during the Qui Dynasty (221-206 B.C.). This contact was intensified by the placement of Chinese military colonies on the northern Korean peninsula during the Han Dynasty (202-220 B.C.). From these contacts, the Korean peninsula was led into a period of rapid advancement in agriculture, health science (which includes the doctrine of the *Nei Ching*), and formalized governmental statesmanship. Confucianism, Taoism, and, later, Buddhism were all introduced to Korea from China.

Due to the advancements in civilization and growing individual tribal unities, three Korean tribal kingdoms were formed: Paekche (18 B.C.), Koguryo (37 B.C.), and Silla (57 B.C.). This was the beginning of what became known as the "Three Kingdom Period" of Korean history.

The Three Kingdoms of Korea entered into a period of continued war against each other and the expansionist Tang Dynasty of China (A.D. 618-907) during the sixth century A.D. This warring period in Korean history instigated the formation of the first group of formally trained and organized soldiers who utilized Ki for other than medical purposes. They were known as the Hwa Rang (Flowering Youth) warriors.

The Hwa Rang warriors were first organized by King Chin-hung of the Korean Kingdom of Silla in A.D. 576. Though his kingdom had its army, his soldiers were believed to be of an unexceptional nature, accounting for his inability, through continued conflicts, to defeat his geographical neighbors, the Koguryo, the Paekche, and the invading Tang Chinese. So King Chin-hung set about organizing a group of talented young noblemen who were exceedingly loyal to the throne, who could be extensively trained in all forms of warfare and then successfully go into battle.

The Kingdom of Silla was based on a Confucian doctrine of society. King Chin-hung believed, however, that the Buddhist canon led to a more calm and pure mind than did Confucianism. To this end, young, hand-some males of Noble birth, some as young as 12 years old, were gathered together. They were dressed in the finest clothing and their faces were attractively painted with elaborate makeup. They were instructed exten-sively in Buddhism (Puk-kyo), medicine (Yak), and the theory of Ki accord-ing to the Nei Ching, and in poetry and song. It was believed that those who fared well in these activities had the divine grace to become superior warriors. A certain number of these young men who excelled were thus recommended to enter the ranks of the Hwa Rang.

These chosen young noblemen were then trained in all known forms of martial combat. As part of this training, they were instructed by Buddhist monks who, through years of meditation, had refined the knowledge of Ki to a point where it was no longer simply a method of rebalancing the Um (Yin) and Yang in the human body. This advanced Ki training taught the young Hwa Rang how to channel Ki energy, first internally to strengthen their bodies against the fierce Korean climate, and then externally in order to become more powerful warriors in battle.

As Buddhism, for the most part, simply passed through China and was not thoroughly absorbed, the Korean peninsula was the first East Asian region to truly accept the doctrine. It was the belief of the Hwa Rang that meditation took place not only in the traditional fashion, in a sitting posture, but was also achievable when individuals focused their personal spirit and then entered into battle with a highly refined purpose and a vision of victory. The battles the Hwa Rang fought thus became spiritual exercises in enlightenment.

The Hwa Rang were the first group of trained warriors ever to pos-sess a spiritual attitude toward warfare. Though the Chinese wrote great philosophic works on warfare, such as The Art of War (Sun Tzu), their focus was on the Confucian concept of political loyalty, not on refined spirituality leading to ultimate enlightenment, as Korean Buddhism taught. This spiritual warrior code developed by the Hwa Rang was first passed on to Japan in the sixth century A.D. From this the famed Samurai tradition was eventually born.

Once a Hwa Rang was fully trained, he was put in command of a military troop composed of several hundred common soldiers. The battles won by the Hwa Rang brought about the unification of Korea. History would not be served, however, if it were not acknowledged that this unification was achieved by very bloody conflicts in which a large percentage of the Korean population was killed.

After the unification of Korea and the defeat of the invading Tang Dynasty, the mind of the Korean people rapidly began to shift from conflict to more philosophic thoughts. As warriors, the Hwa Rang fell into decline by the end of the seventh century. Their refined knowledge of Ki and its healing abilities caused them to become known as a group specializing in Buddhist philosophy, healing, and poetry. No longer, however, did they maintain the high status of royal warriors.

• Ancient Japan •

From the Korean kingdom of Paekche, Chinese philosophic ideals were first transmitted to Japan by King Kunch-ogo (A.D. 346-375). Two Korean scholars, A-Chikki and Wang-In, were sent to Japan to instruct the Japanese Crown Prince in the Confucian doctrines. They brought with them ten copies of the *Analects of Confucius* and one copy of the *Chien Cha Wen* (*The Thousand Character Classic*). This first exposure to Confucian thought proved to be one of the most influential cultural events in ancient Japanese history.

From this initial cultural awakening emerged a group of rulers from the Yamato plain in the southern region of the main Japanese island of Honshu. These rulers, influenced by the concepts of Chinese statesmanship, claimed descent from the Sun Goddess and achieved the first known political unity for Japan by the mid-fourth century A.D. This was the beginning of the Yamato Period in Japanese history.

Buddhist monks were sent to Japan from the Korean state of Paekche in the sixth century to introduce Buddhism to the island nation. The Buddhist monk Kwall-uk (*Kanroku* in Japanese) crossed the Sea of Japan in A.D. 602, bringing with him a large number of Buddhist sutras, historical books, medical books, and works on astronomy, geography, and the occult arts. Kwall-uk was instrumental in the founding of the Sanron school of Buddhism in Japan.

As there was no evidence of Chinese medical practices in Japan until this period, it is believed that this is when the knowledge of Ki, as detailed in the *Nei Ching,* was first transmitted from Korea to Japan. Though Chinese and Korean medicine rapidly expanded throughout Japan and was practiced by monks and priests from this time period forward, the use of Ki for other than medical purposes did not evolve in Japan until the 12th century, with the advent of the Samurai.

The medieval Samurai were military retainers, who, for the most part, were illiterate, rural landowners who farmed between battles. Samurai involvement in government began in 1156. Eventually, the Samurai emerged as military aristocrats and later as military rulers.

In the Gempei War (1180-85), the ruling Taira family was displaced in Japan by the Minamoto clan. Minamoto no Yoritomo (1147-1199) established the first military government, leading Japan into its Kamakura Period (1192-1333) by establishing the Kamakura Shogunate. This was a period of Japanese history in which the aristocratic Samurai governed the country with military rule.

The eldest son of Minamoto no Yoshimitsu, Yoshikiyo, moved away from the central clan to an area known as Kai. Once there, he founded a new branch of the Minamoto clan, known as Kaigengitakeda; Kai from the region, Gengi from the original Chinese root of their family name, and Takeda as the new chosen family name. Thus was born the Takeda family. Through knowledge gained from extensive interaction with learned Buddhist monks, which they combined with their knowledge of war, the Takeda family advanced the understanding of Ki, bringing it to bear on a physical level. This merging of Buddhist philosophy and military lore later gave birth to such martial art systems as Daito Ryu Aikijitsu, Aikido, and Korean Hapkido. All of these modern martial art systems use the principles Ki as their primary basis of physical and mental self-defense awareness.

Today, Ki is used as a healing tool as well as a method in which the individual may gain superior physical prowess and come into contact with universal energy.

Part II

☯

The Meridians:
Passageways of Ki

UNDERSTANDING THE MERIDIANS

K i flows through the human body via what are known as meridians (*Kyung*). Meridians are channels or highly defined pathways inside the human form along which Ki travels. They function in a way very similar to blood vessels, yet they cannot be seen when the human body is dissected. Meridians exist on an ethereal level beyond the physical vision of human beings.

Each organ of the human body has a meridian which governs the flow of Ki to and from it. When an individual's *Um* (Yin) and Yang are in balance, the meridian channels are open and Ki nourishes the organs and the various body functions which they each affect. When an individual's *Um* and Yang are out of balance, the body begins to show symptoms of physical and emotional illness. These symptoms indicate that one or more of the meridians has become blocked.

As was first detailed in ancient Chinese and Korean medical manuscripts and is now confirmed by modern medical science, each of the body's organs handles a specific body function as well as many of the organs' secrete hormones which lead to overall emotional and mental health. Therefore, both physical and emotional health are directly affected by the body's organs.

There are a total of twelve primary or "Constant" Meridians (*Pu-dan-ui Kyung*) in the human body. These twelve meridians are referred to as

"Constant" Meridians because Ki energy circulates through them in a constant and continual delineated path. Ten of these meridians are defined by and govern specific organs of the human body: the Gall Bladder Meridian, the Liver Meridian, the Lung Meridian, the Large Intestine Meridian, the Stomach Meridian, the Spleen/Pancreas Meridian, the Heart Meridian, the Small Intestine Meridian, the Bladder Meridian, and the Kidney Meridian. The final two Constant Meridians—The Heart Constrictor Meridian and the Triple Warmer Meridian—are related to the general control of bodily functions. The Heart Constrictor Meridian dominates the continual flow of blood throughout the body and the Triple Warmer Meridian controls the energy of respiration.

Each of the Constant Meridians is located on both the right side and the left side of the body. Ki flow along the meridians is, therefore, exactly directed to those specific regions of the body the meridian affects. Furthermore, when an individual is experiencing a blockage of Ki flow along any of the Constant Meridians, exacting stimulation can be applied to reinstate proper Ki current. (For the purpose of the simplified illustrations in this text, the individual meridian channels have been depicted on a single side of the human torso, as in figures 3 through 16 in this section).

There are two other meridians which also aid in the control and circulation of Ki throughout the human body. They are the Conceptual Meridian and the Governing Vessel Meridian. These do not possess a direct relationship to a specific body organ and are not an integral element of the body's primary Ki circulatory system, and so they are referred to as Secondary Meridians (*Pu-ch-a-jok Kyung*). These Secondary Meridians influence highly specific Ki channels and bodily activities.

Ki flow through each of the body's meridians progresses in a constant and unchanging direction, either ascending or descending. Each of the meridians is dominated by either *Um* or Yang and possesses one of the five earthly elements previously described.

PRESSURE POINTS

Pressure points (*Hyel*) are precise access sites along a meridian. These *Hyel*, when properly stimulated by acupuncture (*Chim Sul*), acupressure (*Ki-op-sul*), or an exactingly prescribed physical movement, enhance the flow of Ki along a specified meridian.

• Healing Through Pressure Point Therapy •

Hyel stimulation is the method used by acupuncturists and acupressurists to cure any blockage of Ki which may be present in order to rebalance the *Um* and Yang and promote health. By correctly stimulating a *Hyel*, one directs Ki energy to the meridian's organ and all the physical and emotional functions which the specific meridian dominates.

Hyel stimulation does not create Ki in the body. Ki energy is always present in the body. Stimulating a meridian's *Hyel* simply refocuses and redirects additional Ki current along a specific pathway so the body may regain a natural state of balance and health.

Meridian stimulation via *Hyel* is not just a method for healing the body's imbalances. It is also a way to channel additional Ki energy along a meridian when it is known that the functions dominated by the specific meridian are going to be put under extraordinary strain in the coming days. By applying appropriate stimuli to *Hyel* when the *Um* and Yang of the body are in balance, the stimulated Ki will remain present along the exact meridian for approximately twenty-four hours. This time period is, however, governed by the rate of a person's own metabolism. Those who possess very slow metabolisms tend to maintain added Ki flow longer than those who have a faster metabolic rate.

THE MERIDIANS OF THE HANDS

Several of the meridians culminate at the tips of the fingers. The Heart Meridian and the Small Intestine Meridian culminate at the little finger; the Heart Constrictor Meridian culminates at the middle finger with a secondary *Hyel* on the third finger; the Triple Warmer Meridian culminates at the third finger; the Lung Meridian culminates at the thumb; the Large Intestine Meridian culminates at the first finger.

When one uses acupressure to stimulate a *Hyel*, Ki is almost effortlessly passed from the body of the acupressurist into the patient when he or she uses the finger corresponding to the specific meridian. As all meridians do not culminate in the fingers, this type of acupressure massage is only applicable for specific conditions.

TIME IN RELATION TO THE MERIDIANS

Each meridian has a specific time period when it is most active in the natural clock of this Earth. When you are attempting to stimulate Ki flow along a specified meridian, the results are most evident when you perform the treatment in the time period when the Meridian is most active. (See Table 4, page 21).

Table 4. Meridian Timetable.

The Gall Bladder Meridian	12:00 A.M.	to	2:00 A.M.
The Liver Meridian	2:00 A.M.	to	4:00 A.M.
The Lung Meridian	4:00 A.M.	to	6:00 A.M.
The Large Intestine Meridian	6:00 A.M.	to	8:00 A.M.
The Stomach Meridian	8:00 A.M.	to	10:00 A.M.
The Spleen/Pancreas Meridian	10:00 A.M.	to	12:00 P.M.
The Heart Meridian	12:00 P.M.	to	2:00 P.M.
The Small Intestine Meridian	2:00 P.M.	to	4:00 P.M.
The Bladder Meridian	4:00 P.M.	to	6:00 P.M.
The Kidney Meridian	6:00 P.M.	to	8:00 P.M.
The Heart Constrictor Meridian	8:00 P.M.	to	10:00 P.M.
The Triple Warmer Meridian	10:00 P.M.	to	12:00 A.M.

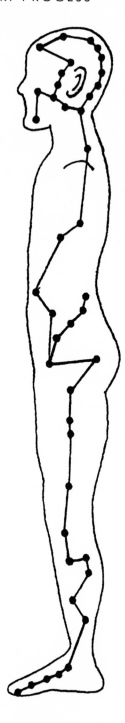

Figure 3. The Gall Bladder Meridian.

THE MERIDIANS

THE GALL BLADDER MERIDIAN
(JOK SU YANG DAM KYUNG)

The Gall Bladder Meridian is Yang. Its element is wood. This meridian has a descending pattern of Ki flow, progressing from the head, down the back of the legs, to the feet (figure 3). Physically, the gall bladder stores and excretes bile to aid in digestion. Mentally, the Gall Bladder Meridian bestows the ability to make clear choices and rational judgments.

If a blockage of Ki exists in the Gall Bladder Meridian, a person may experience digestive problems due to the inability of the body to successfully assimilate one's intake of food. As the Gall Bladder Meridian extends the entire length of the human body, it contacts numerous muscles and tendons. The first signs of Ki blockage in this meridian may be unexplained tension in the back and the neck.

From an emotional standpoint, if Ki blockage exists in the Gall Bladder Meridian, the individual's ability to make rapid, clear, and rational decisions may be impaired. In addition, the individual may be plagued by unexplained negative thoughts.

• Immediate Ki Stimulation of the Gall Bladder Meridian •

Several primary *Hyel* (pressure points) of the Gall Bladder Meridian may be readily accessed at the rear of your head. Reach both hands up and place them in the center of the back of your head. The fingers of your individual hands should be spaced approximately one inch apart. Once your hands have been placed on the back of your head, it is important to not let the fingers of your left and your right hand come into contact with one another as this causes Ki energy disbursement as opposed to Ki energy stimulation. Massage the back of your head with light pressure for approximately three minutes. This will stimulate the pressure points of the Gall Bladder Meridian and cause additional Ki to travel its path.

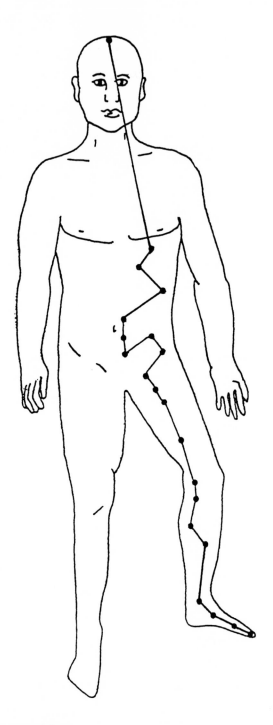

Figure 4. The Liver Meridian.

THE LIVER MERIDIAN (*JOK KWE YUL UM GAN KYUNG*)

The Liver Meridian is *Um*. Its element is wood. The Liver Meridian's Ki flow travels in an ascending path from the feet to a location on the top of the head (figure 4).

From a modern medical standpoint, the liver is the largest glandular organ in the human body. It performs many vital functions, such as the storing of vitamins and nutrients, the purifying of blood, and the secretion of bile in order that the fat in foods which we have eaten may be digested. The liver is easily damaged by the continued drinking of alcohol and coffee.

The liver refines blood and provides it to the rest of the body on demand. When the body is physically active, the liver functions at a higher level, providing larger amounts of blood than when the body is resting or in a state of idleness due to lack of exercise. As blood purity and circulation is directly related to the unhampered flow of Ki in the body, it follows that we should engage in a conscious amount of physical exercise each day to keep the body healthy and functioning properly, with an unrestricted flow of Ki moving within it.

The fingernails and toenails are what the Korean Ki practitioner examines to check on the proper functioning of the Liver Meridian. If the nails are brittle and/or yellowish in color, they tell the physician that the individual has a blockage of Ki flow in the Liver Meridian. If the liver is healthy and the Liver Meridian has abundant Ki flow, the nails are strong and moist.

The Liver Meridian is also known to affect tendons and how they meet and interact with the muscles of the body. Tendons are considered reliant on the continual flow of purified liver blood to remain elastic. If the Liver Meridian is blocked and the Ki current is obstructed, the symptoms of random tightness and pain, not caused by excessive physical activity, will be felt in the joints.

The liver and the Liver Meridian are also responsible for the health of the eyes. As the eyes are sight organs which must have a continual source of purified blood to remain healthy, any blockage of blood flow to them can be very damaging.

From an emotional perspective, the Liver Meridian is known to be in control of various aspects of mood. If the Meridian is Ki-starved, the individual can become depressed for no particular reason. If the meridian becomes rapidly impacted with a new and overabundant flow of Ki due to physical stimulation from caffeine or other drugs, the person may become intensely moody, nervous, or may simply become angry for unexplained reasons.

• Immediate Ki Stimulation of the Liver Meridian •

A daily routine of cardiovascular physical exercise naturally aids in cleansing and removing any Ki blockage which may exist along the Liver Meridian.

Added Ki flow can be dispatched along the Liver Meridian by locating the *Hyel* directly on the top of your head. This *Hyel* is virtually a magnet. If you place your middle finger on top of your head to locate it, the finger will be drawn to it. Once you have located it, put a light steady pressure on it for approximately thirty seconds. Then allow thirty seconds to pass with no pressure. Return your middle finger to its position and, while lightly massaging, apply pressure for three natural breath cycles. This technique should be applied three times a day, morning, noon, and at night just before sleep, if the Liver Meridian is experiencing Ki clogging.

THE LUNG MERIDIAN
(SU TAE UM PAE KYUNG)

The Lung Meridian is *Um*. It possesses the element metal. Ki energy travels through the Lung Meridian running in a descending flow from the chest to the thumb (see figure 5, page 28). The Lung Meridian is responsible for the control and the intake of oxygen and the body's absorption of Ki which is obtained from the air.

The amount of oxygen which is taken in through breathing directly affects the amount of physical and mental energy an individual possesses. From a physiological standpoint, additional amounts of oxygen may be absorbed by the human body when a person leads a consciously active life. This is accomplished by daily cardiovascular exercise rather than a sedentary lifestyle. Cardiovascular stimulation supplies the body with additional amounts of oxygen which, in turn, stimulate all the cells in all parts of the human body.

As Ki is absorbed from the air, an active lifestyle directly affects the overall amount of Ki circulating in the body. Though Ki taken in from exercise is not highly directed to specific regions of the body, it, like oxygen, then stimulates all meridians and parts of the body.

The Lung Meridian is the meridian which protects the body from diseases which affect the respiratory tract, such as colds, coughs, emphysema, tuberculosis, and lung cancer. The Lung Meridian also regulates the pores of the skin to aid the body in adapting to and functioning properly in various temperature ranges. Stimulating and strengthening the lungs and the Lung Meridian through cardiovascular physical exercises and Ki exercises (see Part III) will aid in achieving an overall healthier life.

Symptoms of Ki deficiency along the Lung Meridian are: shortness of breath, chronic cough, general lethargy, weak pulse, and a weak, nondynamic voice.

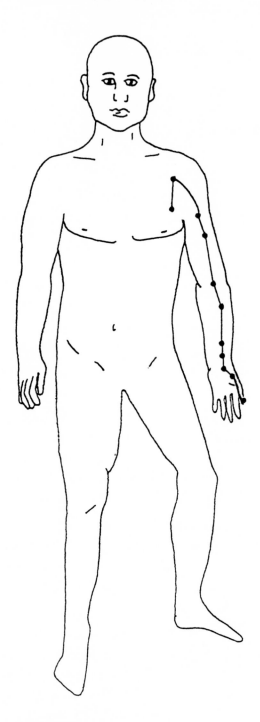

Figure 5. The Lung Meridian.

• Immediate Ki Stimulation of the Lung Meridian •

The Lung Meridian is the easiest meridian to stimulate with Ki energy. As it is directly linked to bodily activity, this meridian can be stimulated simply by taking a fast-paced walk or doing some aerobic exercise that will instantly generate additional amounts of Ki along it.

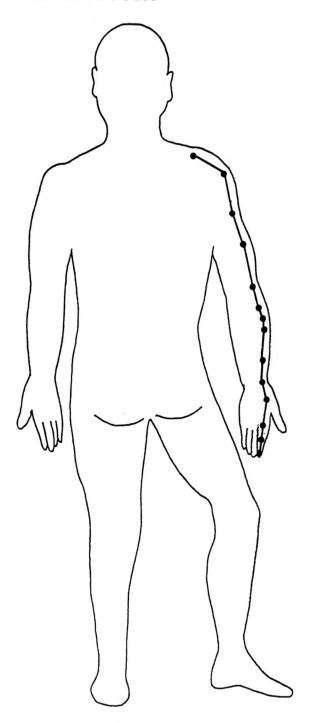

Figure 6. The Large Intestine Meridian.

THE LARGE INTESTINE MERIDIAN
(SU YANG MYUNG TAE JANG KYUNG)

The Large Intestine Meridian is Yang. It belongs to the element of metal. Its path of Ki energy is ascending, traveling from the first finger to the head (figure 6). Physically, the large intestine is responsible for cleansing the body. Emotionally, it controls and expels negative thinking.

The Large Intestine Meridian is responsible for cleansing and detoxifying the human body. In order to achieve this on the physical level, it controls the elimination of solid waste from the body. For people who develop a persistent physical constipation, this signals that the Large Intestine Meridian is blocked and Ki energy is not flowing correctly throughout the meridian.

The Large Intestine Meridian is also in control of the ability to readily cleanse thoughts and emotions. This meridian controls the ability to emotionally "free oneself" or "let go." From the emotional standpoint, if a person becomes highly inhibited and overly reserved, though this is not his or her normal personality, this is a sign that the Large Intestine Meridian is blocked and not allowing a proper flow of Ki.

• Immediate Ki Stimulation of the Large Intestine Meridian •

The primary *Hyel* (pressure point) of the Large Intestine Meridian is located on the hands. This pressure point is directly between the thumb and the first finger, approximately one inch in from the fold of the hand. It is known as *Hap Gok*. By taking the thumb and first finger of your opposite hand and placing light pressure on this *Hyel*, for approximately five natural breaths an hour over a six hour period, the body will obtain relief from physical constipation or unnecessary mental inhibitions.

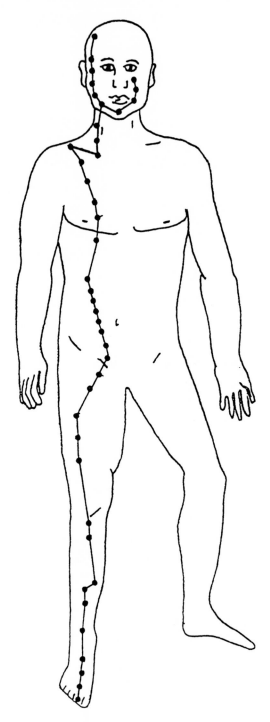

Figure 7. The Stomach Meridian.

THE STOMACH MERIDIAN
(JOK YANG MYUNG WI KYUNG)

The Stomach Meridian is Yang. Its element is earth. Ki energy flows in a descending pattern along it, from the head to the second toe (figure 7). The Stomach Meridian controls the digestion of food.

The Stomach Meridian dominates all forms of digestion in the human body. Foods and liquids first enter the stomach, where they are digested. Specific nutrients are then dispersed to nourish specific regions throughout the body. The stomach is, therefore, one of the primary focal points of human existence. In fact, in ancient Korea, the stomach was thought to be the central organ of the body.

If a person is suffering from digestive problems, the first area of investigation must be diet. A proper diet is the most elemental key to a healthy life. A diet filled with fatty, spicy, and overly sweet foods should be avoided, whereas a natural, high-fiber diet allows the body to function at a superior level. If a person is eating a relatively healthy diet and still experiencing digestive problems, this tells us that the flow of Ki along the Stomach Meridian may be blocked.

• Immediate Ki Stimulation of the Stomach Meridian. •

The Stomach Meridian begins at the upper skull and travels downward along the torso to the second toe. To add additional Ki flow to the Stomach Meridian to aid in the cure of digestive problems, there are two *Hyel* which are of primary importance. They are the *Hyel* in the central temple and the *Hyel* just below the cheek bone.

Take the forefinger and the thumb of both hands and find these pressure points on either side of your face. Put light pressure on them and hold for a period of nine natural breath cycles immediately before and fifteen minutes after you have eaten.

THE SPLEEN/PANCREAS MERIDIAN
(JOK TAE UM BI KYUNG)

The Spleen/Pancreas Meridian is *Um*. Its element is earth. This meridian possesses an ascending flow of Ki energy traveling from the big toe to the chest (figure 8). The Spleen/Pancreas Meridian is responsible for the blood's transformation of food into energy.

In the *Nei Ching*, the spleen is described as the organ which unifies the blood. From a modern medical standpoint, we know the spleen is a highly vascular, ductless organ which modifies, filters, and stores the blood. The spleen creates antibodies such as white blood cells to fight off disease and infection in the human body.

The pancreas is a gland behind the stomach which produces fat-digesting enzymes and the hormone insulin, which the body uses to regulate blood sugar, the source of usable energy. Therefore, the spleen and the pancreas combined allow the body to regulate energy from food and fight off disease.

The body takes sugar and makes it into usable energy in the form of insulin. If the body is continually fed a diet with an overabundance of refined sugar, the body will grow to require unnaturally large amounts of sugar. When this sugar is not constantly present, the body experiences a "withdrawal" from the sugar. This may lead to the medical conditions known as hypoglycemia (low blood sugar) and diabetes mellitus (deficient production of insulin).

Ki flow along the Spleen/Pancreas Meridian is most easily damaged by those who take in large amounts of refined sugars. To avoid this, sugar in the diet should be kept to a minimum. Ideally, sugar should only be consumed in the form of fructose, a sugar found naturally in fruits.

• Immediate Ki Stimulation of the Spleen/Pancreas Meridian •

Though added Ki flow along the Spleen/Pancreas Meridian cannot cure diseases caused by heredity or poor nutrition, stimulating this meridian

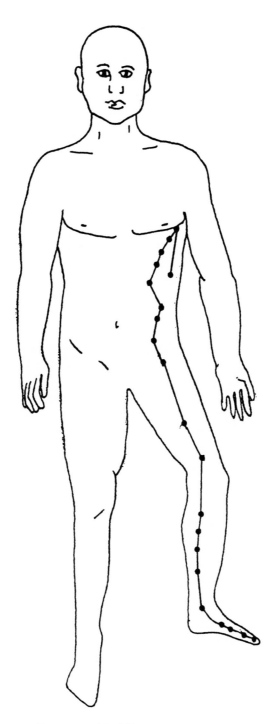

Figure 8. The Spleen/Pancreas Meridian.

can aid in the lessening of some of the symptoms of those diseases. In addition, it can quickly aid those who experience periodic low blood sugar problems and can help the body in the development of additional antibodies when one has an infection or is ill.

To stimulate the Spleen/Pancreas Meridian with additional Ki, first take your hands and place them at your waist with your fingers separated. With your forefingers, feel for the place where the top of your hipbone meets your stomach in the front of your body. Just past this point, where you no longer feel the bone, is a primary *Hyel* of the Spleen/Pancreas Meridian. Apply pressure with your forefinger to these *Hyel* on both sides of your body. As you do, take ten deep yet natural breaths. Allow these breaths to slowly enter and leave your body, as pressure remains on this *Hyel*. This acupressure exercise should be performed once a day.

THE HEART MERIDIAN
(SU SOO UM SHIM KYUNG)

The Heart Meridian is *Um*, with a Ki flow descending from the chest to the little finger (see figure 9, page 38). It possesses the element of fire. The Heart Meridian influences the overall health of the human heart. Therefore, it is very important that this meridian maintain a constant flow of Ki.

From an emotional standpoint, the Heart Meridian affects the consistency of emotions in an individual. If Ki flow along the meridian has become clogged, the person may experience wide mood swings and will become emotionally unstable.

In Korea, the heart is considered the home of the spirit (*Young-hon*). It is therefore the most revered organ. The heart is also one of the organs of the human body most susceptible to damage by both physical and emotional stimuli. The heart can easily become injured in a number of ways: through improper diet, a lack of proper physical exercise, an overabundance of physical stress, emotional trauma, or through a negative psychological approach to life. Though most cases of inappropriate lifestyle can be altered by the individual, people often choose not to change their physical habits or mental approach because of environmental, cultural, or psychological conditioning. For this reason, the heart is most often the first organ of the human body to experience unnecessary damage.

The heart regulates the flow of blood throughout the body. If this organ becomes impaired in any way, all functions of the body's metabolism are adversely affected. The heart and its health should, therefore, be foremost in the mind of the individual.

The Heart Meridian keeps the flow of Ki to the heart constant. If this meridian becomes blocked, the heart will have less ability to fend off the strains of daily life.

To aid the Heart Meridian in remaining clear, one should eat a low-fat diet and partake of regular physical exercise. In addition, one should

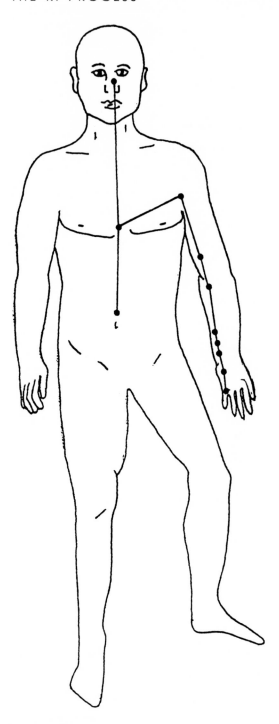

Figure 9. The Heart Meridian.

learn methods such as controlled breathing techniques and meditation to release negative emotional states of mind (see Part III).

• Immediate Ki Stimulation of the Heart Meridian •

The Heart Meridian flows from the chest to the little finger on both sides of the body. Stimulation of the Heart Meridian takes place immediately by applying pressure to its *Hyel* in the fold of your elbow.

To locate this *Hyel*, bend your elbow to a thirty-five degree angle. Reach your opposite hand across and, with your thumb, locate the center of the inside of your elbow crease. You will feel a tight muscle mass. This is your biceps muscle. Move your thumb downward, approximately one eighth of an inch away from this muscle, in the direction of your lower arm. You will feel a slightly soft spot where there is no muscle or bone. This is the *Hyel* of the Heart Meridian. By alternating between light pressure and a light massage for three minutes, your Heart Meridian will experience added Ki stimulation. Repeat the same process on the opposite side.

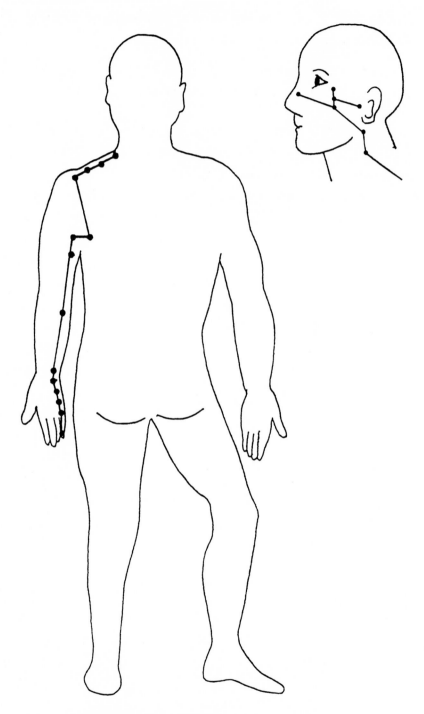

Figure 10. The Small Intestine Meridian.

THE SMALL INTESTINE MERIDIAN
(SU TAE YANG SOO JANG KYUNG)

The Small Intestine Meridian is Yang with an ascending flow of Ki energy traveling upward from your little finger to the base of your neck (figure 10). It has the element of fire. Physically, the Small Intestine Meridian controls the absorption of nutrients into the body from food. If a person is eating a wholesome diet but still feels unduly spent in times of physical activity, blockage of this meridian may be the cause.

Mentally, the Small Intestine Meridian is responsible for the cognitive understanding of newly experienced thoughts and ideas. To an individual who becomes overwhelmed when introduced to new thoughts and ideas, or who does not readily comprehend explanations, blockage of Ki flow along the Small Intestine Meridian may be the cause.

• Immediate Ki Stimulation of the Small Intestine Meridian •

The Small Intestine Meridian runs along the arm. To stimulate the flow of Ki to this meridian, stand in a natural posture. Tense the muscle of your right arm slightly, as you lift it directly out to your side until it is parallel to the ground. As your arm rises, take a deep breath in through your nose. Once you have reached your final position, let the breath out as you guide your arm slowly back down to its original natural position at your side. Perform the same technique with your left arm. Do this three times on each side to substantially stimulate the Ki along your Small Intestine Meridian.

THE BLADDER MERIDIAN
(JOK TAE YANG BANG KWANG KYUNG)

The Bladder Meridian is Yang. Its element is water. It possesses a descending Ki flow running from the head to the foot (figure 11).

Modern medical science teaches us that the bladder receives body waste from the large intestine, the small intestine, and the kidneys, and then disposes of them as urine. This process affects the climate of the entire body. If the bladder is inhibited in any way and not receiving and disposing of these wastes, the natural cleansing of the body cannot take place, and disease results. The Bladder Meridian is, therefore, responsible for the overall balance of fluid levels in the body. If the body's fluid levels are incorrect or unstable, this affects virtually every other aspect of human functioning.

The Bladder Meridian regulates the overall temperature of the body by keeping the fluid level constant and correct. If Ki flow along the Bladder Meridian becomes blocked, the individual may become ill due to internal waste build-up. The first symptoms of this are an unexplained low-grade fever. This is due to the fact that the body's temperature increases when its wastes are not readily expelled.

The bladder can be set into a state of imbalance by two means. Problems can arise when an individual continually partakes of an over-abundance of highly acidic liquids such as citric juices, coffees, dark teas, or dark colas. These liquids have a cumulative destructive effect, not only on the bladder, but on many other internal organs as well. The bladder is also negatively affected if an individual does not drink enough water on a daily basis. Thus, the wastes of the system become stagnant and are not readily cleansed from the body. The initial remedy for any physical bladder problem is to drink in excess of ten glasses of water a day. In this way the bodily systems are continually flushed and cleansed.

The Bladder Meridian is the meridian most sensitive to negative emotional stress and pressure. The Bladder Meridian is understood to develop Ki blockage not only from the unsuitable dietary habits previous-

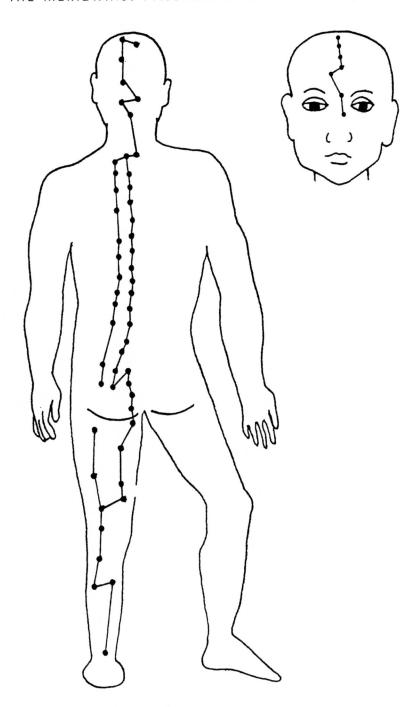

Figure 11. The Bladder Meridian.

ly discussed, but also from the state of bodily disharmony which comes about due to extended periods of emotional strain.

As is often described, emotional pressure is experienced as a stiffness or a pain in the neck or the upper back. The Bladder Meridian's pathway runs directly through the back and the neck. Its *Hyel*, when stimulated, thus has a curative effect, not only by relieving stress but by regulating bodily functions as well. This is why a neck massage feels so good during times of pressure.

• Immediate Ki Stimulation of the Bladder Meridian •

In the event there is no one to provide a neck and back massage (by which even the untrained hand will stimulate the *Hyel* of the Bladder Meridian), the first step in Bladder Meridian stimulation is to get your neck and back moving. This is easily accomplished by simply moving your neck in a circular motion. Once you have moved your neck around several times, activating blood and Ki circulation, you should then stretch it. This is accomplished by bringing your chin in toward your chest. Hold it there for a moment or two, then lean your head back as far as it will go. At this point, stretch it forward and then back one more time. Now stand up if you can; if not, remain seated. Extend your upper arm outward, parallel to the ground. Leave your elbows bent at a ninety-degree angle and rotate your shoulders. With your arm still extended, pivot your upper back from side to side, until you can feel it loosening.

These are just a few examples of how to stimulate Ki flow along the upper Bladder Meridian. In the case of this meridian, any type of comfortable upper body movement will enhance circulation and thus Ki flow.

Once you have loosened your upper body, it is a good idea to drink at least one full glass of fresh water rather quickly. In this way, the physical elements of your bladder will also be stimulated, leading to overall enhanced Ki flow along the Bladder Meridian.

THE KIDNEY MERIDIAN
(JOK SU UM SHIM KYUNG)

The Kidney Meridian is *Um*. Its element is water. Ki travels along the meridian in an ascending pattern, from the heel of the foot to the neck (figure 12).

The kidneys are two separate yet equal functioning organs which continually interact. The kidneys are located at the back of the abdominal cavity. Physically, they are responsible for regulating the acidity in the body and the composition of body fluids. They filter the blood and excrete waste products as urine.

There are two leading causes of kidney malfunction: the continual intake of alcohol over many years, and eating a diet high in salt. Both of these cause destruction of kidney tissue.

According to ancient Korean manuscripts, the kidneys were considered the storage units of the human body. They gathered and stored energy from the blood. This energy was then believed to be released when specific areas of the body needed it. In ancient manuscripts, the kidneys were also linked to an individual's sexual prowess. If a person possessed a healthy sexual appetite, Ki flow along the Kidney Meridian was good. If one experienced sexual tedium, Ki flow along the meridian is blocked.

Though adding Ki flow to a previously damaged kidney cannot reverse the injury, it can aid in the control of overall symptoms of such diseases as cirrhosis. However, if a person is experiencing a lack of physical or sexual energy, or an unexplained blockage of urine flow that a medical doctor cannot cure, the Kidney Meridian may well be blocked. In this case, Kidney Meridian stimulation will be very beneficial.

• Immediate Ki Stimulation of the Kidney Meridian •

The Kidney Meridian culminates at the center of your throat. Place your middle finger in the center of your throat. Follow the indentation of your

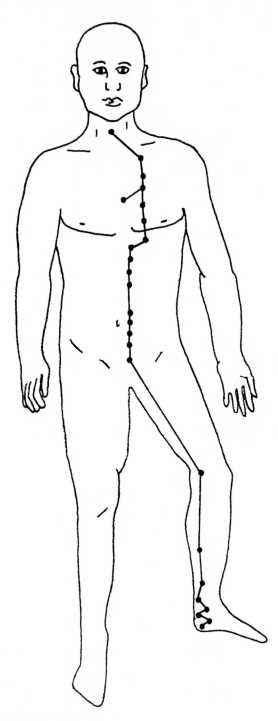

Figure 12. The Kidney Meridian.

throat down until you feel the beginning of your collar bone. At this location is a primary *Hyel* for the Kidney Meridian. Close your eyes and breathe naturally, as you place light pressure on this *Hyel*. Rotate your finger slowly for three natural breaths, then remove your finger. Allow the *Hyel* to emanate Ki for three more natural breaths, then perform the rotating touch again for an additional three breaths. Follow this with a three-breath rest period and then perform the acupressure one more time. This should be performed two times a day, morning and night, until any Ki blockage along the Kidney Meridian is cleared.

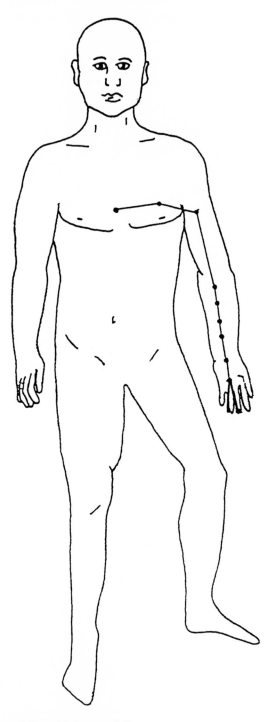

Figure 13. The Heart Constrictor Meridian.

THE HEART CONSTRICTOR MERIDIAN
(SU KWYEL UM SHIM PO KYUNG)

The Heart Constrictor Meridian is *Um*. Its element is fire. Its Ki flow is descending, traveling from the chest to the middle finger, with a secondary *Hyel* on the third finger (figure 13).

The heart regulates the flow of blood throughout the body by means of contraction followed by dilation. The Heart Constrictor Meridian dominates these movements of the heart muscle. Those who experience inconsistent heartbeats can look to this meridian for aid. In addition, individuals who have experienced heart attacks due to poor physical conditioning or stress should also concentrate on adding Ki flow to this meridian, as it directly aids in reestablishing correct heart function.

This meridian becomes clogged and negatively affected (as does the Heart Meridian) by an inactive lifestyle and a high-fat, high-sugar diet.

• Immediate Ki Stimulation of the Heart Constrictor Meridian •

The Heart Constrictor Meridian is positively affected by conscious cardiovascular physical activity. Another method of direct Heart Constrictor Meridian stimulation is to first locate the knuckle of your middle finger with your opposite hand, embracing both the top and the palm of your hand. Once you have located the knuckle, slowly move to the point where the handbone which dominates this knuckle begins. This is the location of the Heart Constrictor *Hyel*. For nine natural breath cycles, firmly massage this location with your thumb and forefinger. This can be performed up to five times a day for Ki stimulation along this meridian.

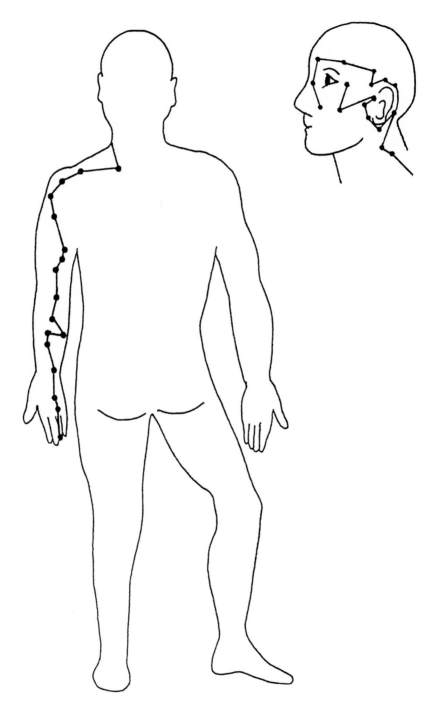

Figure 14. The Triple Warmer Meridian.

THE TRIPLE WARMER MERIDIAN
(SU SOO YANG SAM CHO KYUNG)

The Triple Warmer Meridian is Yang, with an ascending flow traveling from the third finger of the hand to the head (figure 14). Its element is fire.

Ki flow along the Triple Warmer Meridian dominates three specific functions of the body: the energy of respiration, the control of digestion, and the control of body discharge (waste elimination and the discharge of sexual fluid). The *Hyel* which access and add Ki flow to these functions are located in three specific locations on the body: the Upper Level from shoulder to head, the Mid Level from lower shoulder to forearm, and the Lower Level from forearm to hand. Thus, "Triple Warmer."

The Triple Warmer Meridian, when viewed as a whole, has the function of controlling the body's overall temperature. This is because the three separate bodily functions it links (respiration, digestion, and elimination) have a cumulative affect on overall health, and thus on the temperature, of the human body. If any one part of the Triple Warmer Meridian is not functioning correctly, meridian stimulation should be applied.

The Triple Warmer Meridian is also considered to affect the equilibrium of the body. When Ki flow is clogged along this meridian, the individual may experience dizziness and be continually "off balance" or clumsy.

• Immediate Ki Stimulation of the Triple Warmer Meridian •

The Triple Warmer Meridian can be stimulated by locating a primary *Hyel* on the forearm. Progressing upward toward your elbow, find the point one third of the way up the central outside portion of your forearm. Take the third finger of your opposite hand and locate the *Hyel*. Press the location nine times firmly, allowing the pressure to impact the *Hyel* for ten seconds each time. Perform the same meridian-stimulation technique on the opposite arm. Do each arm a maximum of three times a day.

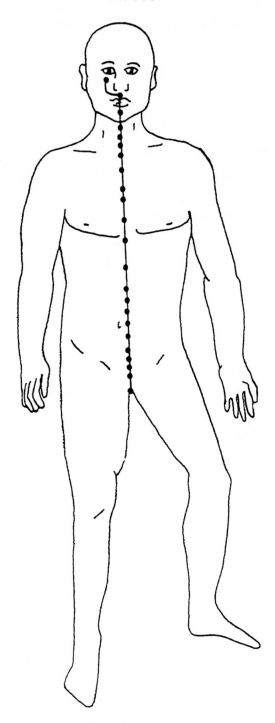

Figure 15. The Conceptual Meridian.

THE CONCEPTUAL MERIDIAN
(IM MACK KYUNG)

The Conceptual Meridian is a Secondary Meridian, not directly linked to a body organ or responsible for the body's primary Ki circulation. The Conceptual Meridian is predominantly an *Um* meridian, though for certain people it acts under the influence of Yang. In addition, an individual may enter into a period where Yang energy is highly prevalent in the body. At this time, the Conceptual Meridian also takes on the aspect of Yang energy. The Conceptual Meridian's element is fire.

Ki is ascendant in this meridian, traveling from the groin to the face (figure 15, page 000).

The Conceptual Meridian regulates the sexual and reproductive Ki energy in a person. If a person is highly driven sexually, this meridian has an abundance of Ki energy. Conversely, if a person is not sexually interested, the Ki flow along this meridian is slow or blocked.

A woman's reproductive cycle is highly affected by Ki energy along the Conceptual Meridian. This meridian, in association with the body's natural clock, sets the timeframe for possible time periods of conception. If Ki flow is blocked along this meridian, a woman may have trouble becoming pregnant.

As sexual and reproductive energy is highly emotional by its very nature, the stability of Ki flow along this meridian directly affects an individual's moods and temperament.

• Immediate Ki Stimulation of the Conceptual Meridian •

Ki flow along the Conceptual Meridian is directly stimulated by concentration on the *Tan Jun* or Center Point (refer to the exercises discussed in Part III).

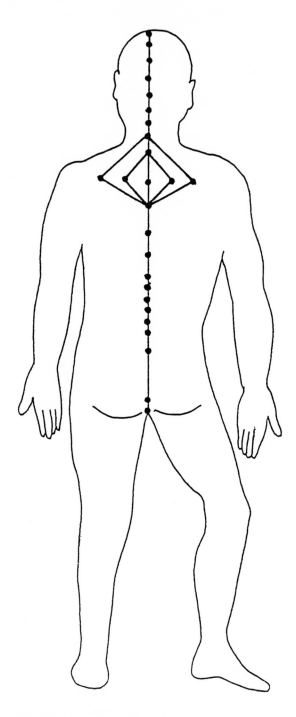

Figure 16. The Governing Vessel Meridian.

THE GOVERNING VESSEL MERIDIAN
(DONG MACK KYUNG)

The Governing Vessel Meridian is a Secondary Meridian acting primarily on Yang energy. *Um* energy does, however, affect and control its functioning during certain individual time periods. A person who is highly *Um*-dominant may find this meridian is continually under the control of *Um* energy. The Ki energy flow along this meridian is ascendant, completely encompassing the upper torso of the body, from the groin, along the spine, over the top of the head, and back down the front of the body to its point of origin (figure 16).

The Governing Vessel Meridian is responsible for balancing the overall functioning of the body. This task is performed by Ki energy continually circulating along this meridian, nourishing and aligning other meridians.

Blockage of Ki along this meridian can occur due to improper diet, consumption of alcohol or drugs, smoking, physical inactivity, or emotional upheaval. If this occurs, all functions of the body will become unbalanced. To prevent this, conscious diet, physical activity, and meditation must be mainstays of your lifestyle.

The first signs of the Governing Vessel Meridian experiencing Ki blockage can be seen on the emotional level. The symptoms are unexplained nervousness, fluctuating mood swings, timidity, unexplained fear, and anxiety.

• Immediate Ki Stimulation of the Governing Vessel Meridian •

To rapidly take control of imbalance in the Governing Vessel Meridian, first stop the intake of any food or liquid which you know to be bad for your health. These may include spicy foods, fatty foods, sugar-ridden foods, coffee, dark teas, dark colas, and alcohol.

Immediately begin a program of physical exercise. This can be as easy as walking fast enough to work up a large amount of perspiration

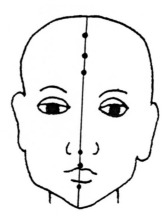

Figure 16. The Governing Vessel Meridian, continued.

every day. As modern medical science now explains, and Korean physicians have known for centuries. During conscious physical activity, the body releases hormones which stimulate physical and mental well-being. This physical exercise will help the body to achieve a natural state of balance.

To effectively access the *Hyel* of the Governing Vessel Meridian, separate your thumb and your first finger. Place your thumb just below your nose. To guide your thumb to the *Hyel*, allow it to follow the cartilage which separates your nostrils to the place where your face begins. This is the first *Hyel*. Now, with your first finger, locate your "Third Eye." This *Hyel* is between the eyebrows approximately one-eighth of an inch up. This *Hyel* is very magnetic. Your finger will be drawn to it. Place equal pressure on both of the *Hyel* and maintain it for nine natural breath cycles. This pressure-point stimulation can take place three times a day: morning, noon, and before sleep.

ACUPUNCTURE

In ancient Korea, bone chips and bamboo slivers were used for acupuncture needles (*Chim*). As time progressed and various types of metals were refined, the belief developed that specific metals led to superior types of Ki healing. This belief system has continued, in some circles, even to the present day.

Gold (*Kum*) is believed to be composed of highly Yang materials. Therefore, gold needles are used to help in the healing of Yang-deficient diseases. Silver (*Un*) is said to be formed primarily of *Um* components. Needles made of silver are thus used to aid in the refocusing of *Um* in the human body.

As human understanding of infection and how it is introduced into the body has expanded through time, the use of acupuncture needles made of unsterilizable metals, such as the ones listed above, has been frowned upon by the scientific community. Today, all acupuncture needles are made of the highest grade surgical steel. Thus, the risk of infection has dropped dramatically in all forms of acupuncture.

It must be understood that acupuncture should never be attempted by an untrained individual. Acupuncture students train for many years to learn the skills necessary to be a proficient acupuncturist. By attempting to perform unskilled acupuncture, not only may your attempt lead to skin infections or internal bleeding; you may, in fact, cause Ki flow to be disrupted further, leading to additional problems of *Um* and Yang imbalance. Acupressure, on the other hand, is quite safe and helpful, and may be performed by anyone with the most basic of skills.

Acupuncturists, acupressurists, and martial artists have trained in precisely locating *Hyel* for centuries. This training is undertaken to master the knowledge of Ki flow. Thus, the Ki practitioner may direct added Ki energy to a specific meridian when necessary, resulting in immediate healing, or in the case of the martial artist during battle, he may deliberately strike one of his opponent's *Hyel* in order to interrupt the adversary's flow of Ki.

Part III

The Mastery of Ki

PRACTICAL APPLICATIONS

*O*nce you understand how Ki energy flows through your body via the meridians and how to keep your body healthy and in harmony with it, you can take the next step in Ki understanding and begin to consciously focalize Ki into specific regions of your body for added physical and mental control. The process of exacting Ki focalization is known as *Ki Gong* and is divided into two sections: *Wae Gong*, which focalizes the power of Ki energy to specific locations in the body, and *Shin Gong*, which allows the individual to develop superior mental powers.

FOCALIZED KI ENERGY

It is imperative that any advanced practice of Ki focalization be undertaken only by Ki practitioners who are highly conscious of the specific results that are desired. In the practice of Ki energy development, focused thoughts and defined goals are paramount, for Ki is a highly refined energy. If its practice is not profoundly focused, all results will be minimal, if in fact there are any results at all.

KI INHIBITING FACTORS

There are two primary physical factors which can prevent the conscious mastery of Ki: improper diet and bodily disharmony. Both of these factors lead the body to inhibit the natural flow of Ki, preventing both the conscious movement of Ki throughout the body and the external emanation of Ki.

DIET AND KI

As we learned in Part II and the study of meridians, diet directly affects Ki flow throughout the body. The type of food commonly consumed and the pattern of eating habits directly affects Ki absorption and expulsion from the body. Improper dietary habits will hinder you from having the ability to consciously focus your Ki energy. For this reason, a healthy diet is imperative in the usage of Ki power. Therefore, as a conscious participant in Ki, you must come to understand the various foods and dietary patterns which will aid or diminish your Ki-focusing abilities.

Meat is a highly Yang food. At times when an individual needs an abundance of Yang energy in his or her body, the consumption of meat is recommended. Conversely, when an overabundance of Yang energy is present in an individual's body, all eating of meat should be avoided.

People who commonly consume large amounts of meat cause their digestive system to become stagnant, as meat takes much longer to digest than do fruits and vegetables. For this scientifically proven reason, meat should not be eaten in overabundance, since a sluggish digestive system may cause both the body and the mind to become lethargic. A constant state of lethargy may cause the Ki flow in the body to be hampered. Moreover, the mind may not be sharp enough to observe this condition in time to rectify it before various meridians become clogged, requiring additional Ki-cleansing methods to repair them so that Ki energy can once again flow through the body unabated.

An individual who continually overeats is also left with a sluggish body and mind. Overeating causes the digestive system to perform its digestive functions constantly. The digestive system is, therefore, not allowed the necessary time to be inactive. This causes Ki energy to be unnecessarily focused on this region of the body so that the direction of Ki to other locations, inside or outside of the body, is hampered.

Individuals who make a habit of eating within three hours before they go to sleep also unnaturally disrupt the processes of their digestive system and interrupt their sleep. By doing this, the digestive system is forced to work when it should be at rest with the remainder of the body. Since the body is constantly at work, it is constantly tired and the natural Ki flow is disrupted.

Foods which possess sugar or caffeine also affect Ki. As physical and mental functions are altered by the stimulating nature of these two products, Ki flow to and from the body is modified. Once these two products have been consumed, it takes many hours, and in some cases days, for their overall effects to completely disappear from the human body. In the meantime, Ki mastery is hampered as the physical body and mind are forced to deal with their physiological effects.

Sugar is an *Um* substance. As in the case of meat, it can be consciously utilized to enhance the presence of *Um* in the body when necessary. When it is eaten without necessity, however, it does much more damage than good. In the same way, caffeine can be used as a direct method to enhance alertness. Its components are, however, physically addicting and, due to the highly acidic nature of caffeine and such products as coffee, colas, and dark teas in which it is found, the continual intake of caffeine can physically damage the body. Any benefits caffeine offers are therefore overshadowed by its negative physical consequences.

The trends of modern society have left many individuals seeking the slimmest waistline possible. Undereating, however, leaves the body and mind starved for nutrients, which, in turn, does not allow Ki to progress naturally along the meridians. Avoidance of meat and sugared foods, combined with a diet possessing a full variety of fruits, vegetables, and grains, leaves the body healthy and body fat at a minimum.

BODY DISHARMONY AND KI

The body is set into a state of disharmony when it is strained excessively either through physical or mental means. Body disharmony inhibits the natural flow of Ki, thus creating additional physical and mental problems. If a person exists in a state of bodily disharmony, mastery of Ki is not possible.

It is very common in modern society for people to stress their body excessively without ever realizing that it is taking place. This propels the body into a state of disharmony, while at the same time it continually seeks compensating methods for recovery.

Physical and mental disharmony are caused by such factors as a poor diet, a strenuous work schedule, an overly aggressive exercise program, lack of daily relaxation, or lack of sleep due to any number of reasons. From a biological standpoint, disharmony can occur from the use of alcohol or drugs, even those which are prescribed by a physician.

There are many random elements in this life which are unpredictable. Those who desire to maintain balance and harmony in their lives must choose to deliberatly and consciously perform a regemin of precisely defined physical and mental activities. Any activity you undertake must be accomplished with a completely conscious understanding of what that activity entails. No longer should you simply witness life happening to you and return home tired, injured, discouraged, or disabled from the experience. By consciously embracing and interacting with life, the body and mind will be allowed to maintain a continual state of harmony.

To enter into the path of Ki means that you choose to take conscious control over the elements which inhabit the universe around you. You must, therefore, first maintain a mastery over the physical aspects of your life which are, in fact, much easier to understand and control than Ki energy is. As a result of this simple self-mastery, bodily disharmony will not affect you, and your path to Ki development will be unhindered.

THE FIVE STATES OF KI

As you become a conscious participant in Ki energy, you will rapidly develop the ability to consciously control the five distinct states of Ki: *Kyung Ki* (Light Ki), *Jung Ki* (Heavy Ki), *Chyel Ki* (Firm Ki), *Ma Ki* (Devoid of Pain Ki), and *Shin Ki* (Mental Ki). As you consciously work with the various states of Ki energy you will readily develop the knowledge that allows you to alter the flow of Ki in the body and to achieve the desired state of body and mind.

Ki energy is available to everyone. In the following pages you will be instructed in specific techniques which any individual can safely practice—techniques based in ancient Ki-focalizing methods. The results depend only on your dedication and on your ability to gradually focus and refine Ki energy in your body. Through Ki mastery, you can rapidly achieve enhanced health and energy, as well as a clearer understanding of how we are all integral parts of this everflowing energy-filled universe.

THE FOUR BASIC PRINCIPLES OF KI

There are four basic principles which must be consciously practiced in order to master Ki:

• Release of all stress from the body •

If the mind is clouded with worldly preoccupations, it can never focus on the higher ideals of body and mind unification and a conscious understanding of Ki. To free the mind from these distractions, the practitioner of Ki utilizes concentration and meditation techniques. Through the use of these techniques, an individual quickly develops the ability to view the fleeting nature of emotions, which come and go. Through this under-standing, the Ki technician has the ability to focus the mind, thereby quickly letting go of negative emotion which can bring about stress and impede the flow of Ki.

• The focus and utilization of Ki originates from the center point (Tan Jun) •

The Center Point (*Tan Jun* in Korean, *Hara* in Japanese) is a location on the human body approximately four inches below the navel. This location is not only the gravitational center of balance of the human body, it is also the location where Ki congregates and is thence dispersed throughout the human form. Through the defined understanding and usage of the *Tan Jun*, the Ki practitioner can come to a superior level of balance and an enhanced ability to receive and transmit Ki.

• The mind is consciously linked with the body •

The average person is completely unaware of a functional link between the body and the mind; the body moves as directed, but its movements possess no conscious purpose. The average person struggles throughout life against his or her own body mass, attempting to move the body and control it in unnatural patterns. Through concentration, meditation, knowledge of the *Tan Jun*, and prescribed physical movements, the Ki practitioner gains a superior control over the natural movement patterns of the body, through understanding how Ki most effectively flows through it.

• The undemanding absorption of Ki •

Ki flows throughout the universe naturally. Those who have a knowledge of its existence and vainly attempt to possess and control it, are over-whelmed and destroyed by its power. The conscious practitioner of Ki, on the other hand, allows Ki to enter his or her body naturally, utilizing it as necessary but not attempting to possess it. The Ki of these individuals then naturally flows outward and continues its natural passage through the universe.

By consciously putting these four basic principles to use in your daily life, you not only come to a refined understanding of how Ki affects the human body, you also immediately experience a more calm self and are able to have a more balanced interaction with the world.

THE HUMAN BREATH

Breath (*sum*) is the source of life. Without breathing, human life instantly ceases. Ki is brought into the body through breath. Therefore, breathing is the primary element of Ki.

Correct breathing is the essential component in the development of Ki. Oxygen taken in through breathing is the force which drives the human metabolism. When large amounts of oxygen are taken into the body, the blood and the cardiovascular system are invigorated and become naturally healthy. The average person, however, breathes incorrectly and does little to stimulate the flow of blood through the body by physical exercise. Therefore, the cardiovascular system becomes sluggish and, with aging, slows down and eventually degenerates, becoming prone to unnecessary disease.

Ancient Korean manuscripts discuss how dirty or polluted blood is the source of all disease. They describe how the blood becomes dirty or polluted by an inactive flow. The inactive flow of blood is brought about by physical inactivity and incorrect breathing, leaving the body starved of Ki.

The first thing anyone on the road to Ki development must do is to understand correct breathing.

• The Natural Breath Exercise •

1. Breathe in naturally. Notice whether your breath is taken in through your nose or your mouth. If the breath is taken in through your nose, this is correct natural breathing. If you are breathing in through your mouth, this is incorrect breathing.

The nose is miraculously designed to filter out many of the impurities which inhabit the air around us. By breathing naturally through the nose, many of these impurities are filtered out before they reach your lungs. If you continually breathe in through your mouth, impurities can travel through your throat and into your lungs unrefined.

If you breathe through your mouth in a natural and relaxed state, you must strive to correct this by very consciously breathing through your nose. Incorrect breathing is a learned behavior; it can therefore be corrected by unlearning the inappropriate technique.

2. Watch your breath as you take it in. Does your stomach expand with the inflow of this breath? If it does, this is correct. If your stomach does the opposite—that is, if it pulls inward with the inflow of breath—this is incorrect breathing.

Allowing your stomach to contract when breath is taken in restricts the flow and the amount of air which can be inhaled. By restricting the inflow of air, you substantially hinder your body's ability to take in oxygen. Thus, your body becomes oxygen-starved and numerous respiratory diseases may occur.

If you find you are breathing incorrectly, consciously extend your stomach as each breath comes in. Several times a day, notice your breathing pattern and consciously correct this old habit, until an expanding abdomen becomes a natural part of your normal breathing pattern.

3. Stand up. Take a breath in naturally through your nose and allow it to fill your lungs as your stomach expands. How deeply does your breath permeate your abdomen?

If you witness a baby breathing, its breath is taken in naturally and its stomach expands all the way down to the pelvic region. If you witness an elderly person, a person who smokes, or one who does little physical exercise, you will notice their breathing is generally very shallow, expanding only the chest. From these examples, we can understand what type of breathing is most natural and beneficial to the human body.

If you find your breath is shallow, begin to inhale consciously through your nose, allowing your lungs to expand as you very deliberately direct your breath to your lower abdominal region. Feel the breath fill your lungs and stomach with life-giving oxygen. Practice this directed breathing technique several times a day, until your breath, again, finds its way deep into your body, giving you longevity, health, and Ki.

If you find you do not breathe in a natural manner, do not mentally chastise yourself. Many people, as children or young adults, develop incorrect breathing techniques. Instead of blaming yourself, view this as an opportunity to make a conscious change for the betterment of your body and to move into a healthier and fully functional temple of your soul.

TAN JUN—THE CENTER POINT

Ki is ever-present in the human form. To develop the ability to tap into large amounts of Ki without meridian pressure point stimulation or physical Ki exercises, you must know about your Center Point, the *Tan Jun* in Korean, the *Hara* in Japanese.

The *Tan Jun* is the body's natural center of gravity. It is also the physical location from which Ki is dispersed throughout the human form. For this reason, this location on the human body is highly revered.

The *Tan Jun* is located approximately four inches below the navel. Around this central location, the *Tan Jun* extends approximately one inch in all directions. Once you have located your *Tan Jun,* you will be able to better isolate and use the movements of your body than the person who has no knowledge of the *Tan Jun.* You will also be able to readily channel and effectively move Ki throughout your entire body.

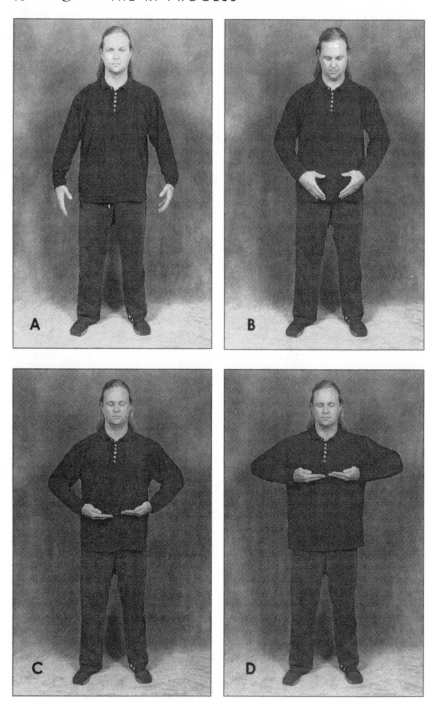

Figure 17. The *Tan Jun* Exercise.

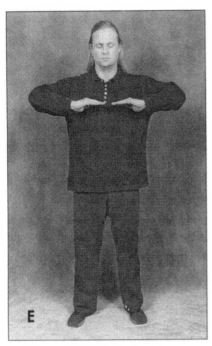
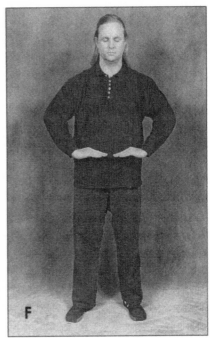

Figure 17 continued.

• Defining Your *Tan Jun* Exercise •

Stand with your legs separated, each approximately even with its respective shoulder. Bend your knees slightly. Your feet should point forward in a natural pattern. Bend your elbows slightly. Extend the fingers of your hand to a naturally straight position. Do not tighten the muscles of your hand, but allow your fingers to be semi-relaxed and naturally separated (see figure 17a). Bring your two hands in front of your *Tan Jun*. Separate your thumbs from your forefingers, allowing them to form an inverted triangle with approximately one inch of separation between your thumbs and forefingers (figure 17b).

Once you have achieved this stance, close your eyes and breathe slowly yet deeply. Allow your breathing to go deep into your abdomen. Once you achieve a relative state of calm, take approximately ten natural breaths and begin to visualize the location of your *Tan Jun* (figure 17c).

Now pivot your wrists until your open palms face upward. Bring your fingers together and allow them to point toward one another. Breathe in deeply through your nose as you visualize your breath entering your body in a golden flow through your *Tan Jun*. As you perform this exercise, bring your hands slowly up your body, following your breath, until they reach your chest level (figure 17d).

Once you have taken in a full breath, hold it in for a moment. Then, as you release it, pivot your palms over to a downward-facing position and allow the breath to leave your body naturally, as your hands travel downward to their original position. As your breath leaves your body, visualize it exiting through your *Tan Jun* in a golden flow (figure 17e,f).

As you perform this exercise, the exact location of your *Tan Jun* will come into clear focus and you will develop the ability to direct Ki easily throughout your body. To effectively develop the ability to readily tap into the Ki energy based in your *Tan Jun*, you should practice this exercise on a daily basis at the onset of your Ki training. Once you have defined a clear focus of your *Tan Jun*, this exercise can be performed whenever you desire to formally clarify the location of your *Tan Jun* or to consciously link yourself with your body's center of Ki.

The *Tan Jun* is the defining factor of overall physical balance in your life. Of course, modern medical science relates many areas of human balance to the inner ear. This notwithstanding, the center of conscious balance for the human body is the *Tan Jun*.

Once you develop a clear awareness and understanding of your *Tan Jun*, you can begin expanding upon this understanding and integrate it into your everyday life through simple techniques. For example, when you move your body from one location to another, begin to take notice of how your *Tan Jun* reacts to your movement. Begin to observe how each movement you make feels in relation to your *Tan Jun*. When you feel off balance, or you lose your balance and slip and fall, how conscious are you of your *Tan Jun*?

By making a conscious effort to concentrate on your *Tan Jun* as you move, you will not only come to a refined level of balance in all of your movements; you will begin to understand how your *Tan Jun* is also your storehouse for Ki energy.

• *Tan Jun* Standing •

How you stand is one of the most important factors in the movement of Ki throughout your body. If you stand with bad posture, slouched over, the upper muscles of your body and the muscles of your legs will continually be fatigued. In addition, you will suffer from unnecessary weakness, as your body is constantly in a state of strain. In terms of equilibrium, you will find yourself continually "off balance," as your spine is not being allowed to encounter the world in the way in which it was designed.

The quickest way to determine if you are standing correctly is to stand up, separate your legs to shoulder width, and allow your arms to fall naturally to your sides. Begin with a posture check. Straighten your spine. How far do you have to extend it upward to achieve an erect posture?

Stand with your spine erect for a moment. Does the straightening of your spine force you to feel uncomfortable after a few moments? If so, this is due to the fact that the lower and middle muscles of your back have been allowed to relax unnaturally over a long period of time. This is the predominant cause of bad posture. If this is the case, consciously put the thought in your mind that you will strive to correct your posture, to become healthier and have a greater flow of Ki through your body. Each time the thought comes to your mind, correct your posture. In a short period of time, this bad habit will have left you, having been replaced by a healthier standing position.

As a second test, ask yourself if you often fidget when you stand. Do you shift your weight from side to side? Do you find it hard to maintain a comfortable standing position? If so, this tells you that your posture is either unnaturally aligned to one side or that your upper body is not in harmony with your lower body.

To test if your spine is misaligned, stand erect, feet at approximately shoulder width, hands naturally at your side. From the base of your spine, allow your upper body to lean slowly—just a few inches—from side to side. Do this a few times. Pause at the place where you feel most comfortable and stop. Is your upper body leaning slightly to one side? If so, this means that, through time, you have developed a bad habit. This is nothing which cannot be corrected, so do not worry about it.

To correct a misaligned spine, perform the previous test two or three times a day—ideally, in the morning when you wake up, at midday, and just before your go to sleep at night. Each time you perform this correction exercise, lean a little farther to each side. Ultimately, allow yourself to lean perhaps a foot to every side each time you do it. This exercise, along with the conscious thought of moving your body into a more natural posture, will cause your spine to realign in a short period of time.

If you find your spine placement is satisfactory, but you still are uncomfortable in a standing position, this tells you that your upper body is not in harmony with your lower body. To correct this, begin by performing the Standing *Tan Jun* Exercise.

• Standing *Tan Jun* Exercise •

Assume a standing position. In bare feet, stand with your knees slightly bent at approximately shoulder width. Consciously keep your spine erect. Allow your back muscles to be as relaxed as possible. Your hands should remain loosely at your side. Allow your eyes to remain open, focused straight ahead (figure 18a).

Lift both of your heels approximately one inch off the ground. Balance yourself on the balls of your feet (figure 18b).

This simple exercise immediately causes your mind to link with your body and form a cohesive unit. Because this body posture, though not difficult, is one most people never assume, it requires conscious thought to maintain the balance necessary to keep your body thus positioned.

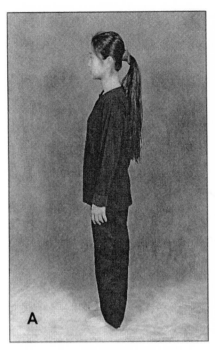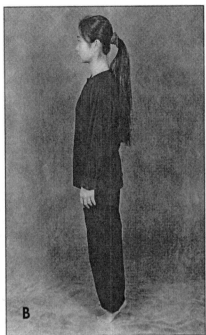

Figure 18. Standing *Tan Jun* Exercise.

As your mind links with your body and you find your natural balance, begin to focus on your *Tan Jun*. After balancing for a moment, allow your *Tan Jun* focus to expand and travel downward along your upper legs. Feel how your legs are an integral part of your body. See them no longer as simply standing or walking tools. Instead, know that they are the driving instruments of your Ki which give you the ability to travel unhindered.

Move your *Tan Jun* focus down a little farther. Feel your knees. Feel the slight bend in them. Notice that it is this slight bend which helps you to maintain your balance in your current stance. Permit yourself to come to a conscious understanding of how these sensitive joints bend and move, balancing your body and propelling you through life.

Once the importance of your legs and knees has been firmly visualized, allow your *Tan Jun* consciousness to travel farther down to your ankles and then out along your feet. Your ankles link you to your feet.

Your feet connect you to the Earth. The Earth is pulsating and alive. It, too, emanates Ki energy. Feel the Ki radiating between your uplifted heels and Mother Earth. Mentally see this exchange of energy. *Ji Ki* is the Korean expression for Ki emanating from the Earth. Feel the balls of your feet and your toes, which touch the ground. Feel the firmness they encounter in the ground below you. Understand how they are the instruments which allow you to impact the ground and move through life.

Mentally see your toes. Extend your mind. Allow yourself to feel each individual toe mentally. The toes are the endpoints of several meridians; feel the Ki energy emanating from them.

Remain standing in this position, coming into mental contact with the lower part of your body, for approximately one minute (or however long you feel comfortable in this stance). Even though you may quickly develop an added sense of balance, perform this exercise often, to link your mind consciously to the importance of your lower body.

In several of the Ki exercises described in this book, you will be asked to stand. Do not, however, allow yourself to stand without conscious awareness of your movements. Instead, enter into your standing position with a full awareness of your lower body and the importance of your legs, knees, ankles, feet, and toes to your overall balance and your personal interaction with universal Ki.

KI BREATHING

Once you have guided your body into a state of correct natural breathing and fully comprehend your *Tan Jun*, you may take the next step in focused Ki development: Ki breathing (*Ki Sum-swi-da*).

Breath control techniques are utilized as a primary method in the development of Ki. Breath control methods are designed to enhance the flow of Ki into your body in the most efficient way possible.

During the Ki-development exercises in the following pages, you will be instructed how to intake, hold, and expel your breath in a prescribed manner to facilitate maximum Ki circulation in each exercise.

Though a variety of Ki breath controls are illustrated in the following pages, there is a single primary method of breath control used in association with Ki development: Four Phase Breath.

• The Four Phase Breath •

The Four Phase Breath, as its name implies, is a four-part breath control technique. In this Ki-focalizing method, you first allow the breath to enter your body through your nose, to pass through your lungs, and to travel on to your *Tan Jun*. The intake of this breath is performed in a continuous manner. It should not be broken up into one or more small spurts, as this will disrupt the flow of Ki into the body.

Once the intake of this breath is complete, allow the air to remain locked in the *Tan Jun* region of your abdomen for a moment. Experience the fullness of your body being embraced with Ki energy. You should not allow small amounts of air to escape little by little, as this breaks up the circulation of Ki in your body.

In the third part of the Four Phase Breath, allow your breath to exit your body in a continuous natural flow. As with the intake, this should be a continuous process, not hindered or broken up by muscle control from your abdomen.

Once all of the oxygen has left your body, allow yourself to remain completely empty of air for a moment. Feel the lightness this creates. When you feel it is time to breathe again, repeat this four phase process.

• Four Phase Breath Exercise •

Settle into a kneeling position. The kneeling position is achieved ceremoniously by first allowing your left knee to slowly drop to the ground, as your right knee bends to accommodate this movement. Then extend your left foot outward behind you and embrace the floor with the top of this foot. Slowly lower your right knee to the ground as your right foot follows

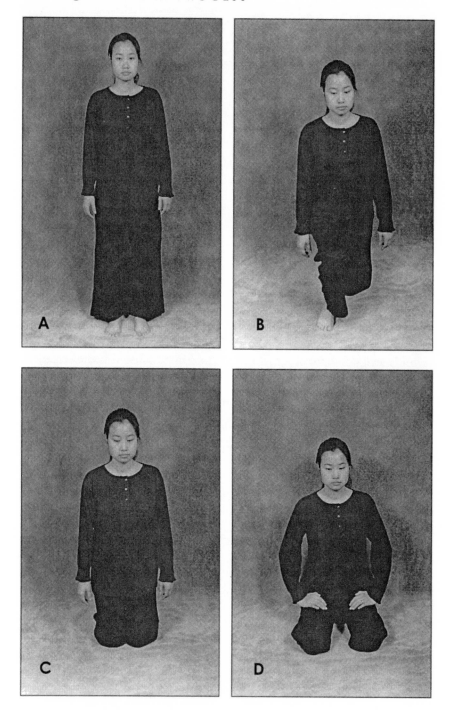

Figure 19. The Four Phase Breath Exercise.

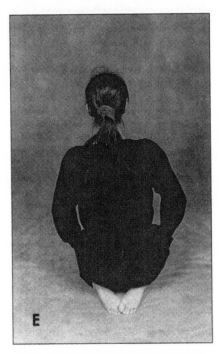

Figure 19 continued.

the same pattern of extending backward. Your knees are left with approximately a one-foot separation between them. Place the big toe of your right
foot on top of the big toe of your left foot and straighten your spine. (See
figure 19.)

This kneeling position has been used in Ki development for centuries, as it forms a firm upward structure and is thus ideal for Ki breathing exercises.

Not everyone can remain seated in this position comfortably for an
extended period of time. If this is the case for you, simply sit in a chair
with your spine erect to perform any of the seated exercises described in
this book.

1. Inhale deeply in a continuous flow though your nose. Allow the intake
of breath to be silent. Never force the intake of breath, as this only causes
resistance from the body, thus creating an imbalance in the flow of Ki.
Visualize the breath entering your body in the form of golden light,

expanding to every part of your torso. Allow the breath to fill your lungs. As the intake of breath is in progress, allow your stomach to expand naturally with the breath's presence. See the breath reaching your *Tan Jun*, illuminating this region.

2. Once your intake of air has been completed naturally, feel its presence remain in the form of golden light throughout your body. See your *Tan Jun* pulsating with the essence of this golden light. Witness your body permeated with golden light, with Ki emanating from all of your pores.

3. Do not allow breath to leave your body in a broken flow. This disrupts the flow of Ki. Allow your breath to exit in a consciously continuous natural motion.

As your breath exits your body, visualize any impurities your body may possess leaving with it. All which remains is pure golden light. Continue this exhalation process until your lungs are completely empty.

4. Once you have exhaled completely, do not attempt to refill your lungs immediately. This may take a bit of practice, for many people panic when they feel empty of oxygen. Instead of immediately inhaling, feel how light your body has become from the absence of air. Observe the emptiness and the purity it possesses. When it becomes time to breathe naturally, do so. Allow the consciousness of Ki to again enter your body.

The Four Phase Breath can be used to enhance Ki visualization and circulation in your body. When you first begin to use this Ki breath-control method, allow each phase to last approximately five seconds, or whatever amount of time feels natural to your body. At the outset, do not attempt to hold any phase longer than feels comfortable. This can cause you to disrupt the natural flow of Ki in and out of your body and may even cause you to pass out. As you continue with the further development of Ki energy via the techniques in this book, you will find that, due to the increased amount of Ki energy circulating throughout your body, the time period of each phase of this breath control will increase, until each phase may last as long as one minute.

As you continue through various exercises in the book, though specific points of oxygen intake and expulsion are described, use this Four Phase Breath as your standard for breath control, as this is the most appropriate type of breathing to use in the development of Ki.

CONCENTRATION (CHIP-JUNG HA-DA)

To achieve any goal, you must be able to firmly focus your mind. But how can you focus your mind if you are surrounded by a world of thoughts, emotions, and objects that you do not truly understand? In this section we will come to understand how you can define your own thoughts, your own body, and your relationship to all things which surround you. From this, you will come to a much clearer understanding of Ki.

The mind of the average person runs from one subject to the next and again the next before he or she even notices this process is taking place. If you desire to achieve your goals, you must stop the process of letting momentary emotions and various stimulating elements of the world drive you from one thought to the next.

• Concentration Exercise 1: Thought Observation •

Sit down comfortably. Close your eyes. Allow your breath to flow naturally, in and out. Allow your mind to think of whatever thoughts come into it. Do not, at this point, judge or attempt to change your thoughts; simply observe each thought as it takes center stage in your mind. Within a few minutes your mind will no doubt have gone from one thought to another. Allow this natural process to take place for several minutes.

There will come a natural point where your conscious mind realizes that your thoughts are racing by. The moment that realization occurs, stop yourself and begin to view how each of the preceding thoughts made you feel. Did some thoughts make you feel agitated and did your heart rate and blood pressure increase? Did other thoughts make you desirous of a person or an object? Did yet other thoughts make you feel calm and relaxed?

Most people, when they allow their minds to "run wild," go through the entire gambit of desires and emotions in a very short period of time. Though this pattern may be a natural occurrence and may at times even be fun, if you allow this type of thought pattern to dominate your life, it will not only waste a lot of your time, but may cause you an enormous amount of grief, as you will lose out on accomplishing many of the things you desire.

• Concentration Exercise 2: Observation Equals Control •

As you prepare to perform this concentration exercise, resolve to let nothing you do be simply random. For example, as you sit down, observe what muscles and joints guide you into this position. Observe the feeling of embracing the chair or the floor with whatever part of your body encounters it. Allow yourself to feel and then savor the sensation of sitting. How does it feel? As you remain seated for a few moments, what type of sensory changes occur in your body and mind?

Close your eyes. How does it feel to close your eyes consciously? What do your eyelids feel like as they come to rest, protecting your eyes?

After observing how your body and mind react for a few minutes, begin to turn your concentration inward. Observe your breath going into your body. How does the oxygen entering your lungs feel? Watch the air as it naturally exits your body. What type of sensation does it create as it leaves?

After observing your breath for several minutes, leave your eyes closed and let your senses reach out from your body and encounter the environment around you. How does the room surrounding you feel? Is it a good feeling? If so, why? Is it a negative feeling? Why? Allow your higher senses, not your eyes or your sense of touch, to explore the walls, the corners, the furniture,

This expansion of your senses is one of the elementary techniques for developing the ability to extend your Ki from your body. For Ki is not defined or influenced by sight. Ki is energy encountering energy.

For most people, life goes by in an instant. They never take the time to witness how their body truly feels or how their surroundings affect them. As science has taught us, all things, be they living plants and animals, or seemingly inanimate objects such as furniture or homes, have a moving energy flowing within them. By fully understanding first how your body feels and then how all the physical elements around you feel, you will have an expanded understanding of internal and external energy and thus a greater knowledge of Ki.

Through the continued practice of this concentration exercise, you will become naturally aware of the sensations present in your body and very conscious of the energy which surrounds you. From this knowledge, you will develop a heightened sense of body consciousness and intuition.

• Concentration Exercise 3: Thought Focusing •

Sit down consciously and close your eyes, as described in Concentration Exercise 2. Observe the feelings of your body and your incoming and outgoing breath. Allow this observation period to last for approximately two minutes. Now send your senses out beyond your body; feel your atmosphere. What energies are present around you? Allow yourself to extend your Ki outward to encounter these external energies for approximately one minute.

Now that you have defined any internal or external stimuli, bring your focus back to your own mind. Begin very consciously to watch your breath enter your body. Feel it go through your nose, travel to your lungs, and then encountering your *Tan Jun*. Now observe the process in reverse. Feel the air exit your body, as it travels up from your *Tan Jun*, through your lungs, and out through your nose.

As breathing is the single most important factor which maintains your life, it is the source of Ki. Consciously explain to yourself that this is why you are performing this concentration exercise: to develop and refine your Ki. As you continue the exercise, see your breath as cosmic energy entering your body from outside, around your body. You then borrow this energy for a time. Witness how this energy leaves your body and expands into the undefined cosmos.

Watch your breath. Observe the Ki entering your body. Visualize your body pulsating with all the continually moving energy of the universe. Feel your separateness fade into the cosmic whole.

Concentration is the first step to meditation. By making the mind devoid of unnecessary thought, you achieve a natural state of meditation.

MEDITATION (MOON-YUM)

Meditation techniques have been handed down since the dawn of time as a means of mental refinement. Meditation is the single most important practice a person can employ to develop an awareness of Ki. As Ki is not a physical strength but a universal energy, the only way one can come into contact with it is through a deepened understanding of the inner working of the body and mind. This understanding is quickly obtained through defined Ki-meditation techniques.

Practitioners of yogic meditation, based in ancient Hindu and Buddhist philosophy, are taught to focus their meditative concentration on *Ajna Chakra*. This is a site of power located between the eyebrows. It is more commonly known as "the Third Eye." The Ki practitioner, however, focuses meditation on his or her *Tan Jun*, thus developing a heightened awareness of Ki, as well as grounding his body to the Earth more efficiently.

• Kneeling Abdominal Breathing Meditation •

To begin this exercise, assume a kneeling posture. As you should not rush immediately into a meditative state of mind, allow yourself to relax and reflect for a moment. When you feel ready, close your eyes and take a deep breath, allowing the air to stimulate your *Tan Jun*. Hold the breath for as long as is comfortable in your *Tan Jun*, then consciously release it (figure 20a and b)

Place your right thumb on your nose and push against your right nostril, closing it off. Breathe slowly yet deeply through the left side of your nose (figure 20c). Observe your breath as it enters and slowly flows to your *Tan Jun* in a golden stream. Once the breath has been taken in fully, allow it to remain for at least five seconds. Now open your right nostril by removing your thumb and at the same time close your left nostril by placing a finger against it. Allow the golden breath to flow naturally

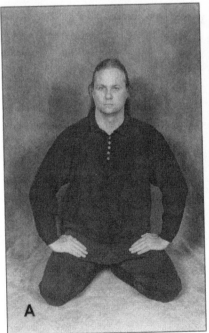
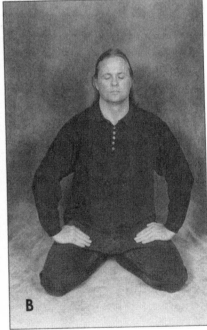

Figure 20. Kneeling Abdominal Breathing Meditation.

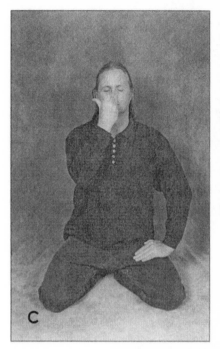

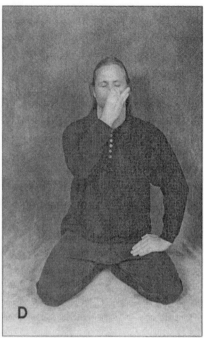

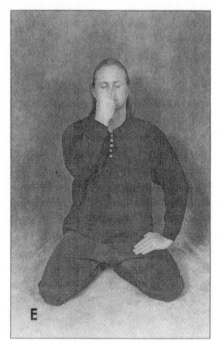

Figure 20 continued.

from your *Tan Jun* out through your right nostril. Once your breath has exited completely, feel the serene emptiness (figure 20d). When it is again time to breathe, take the breath in through your right nostril (figure 20e). Hold it in your *Tan Jun*. When the time of release comes, close off your right nostril with your thumb, opening your left nostril, allowing the breath to exit via your left nostril.

Repeat this process approximately twenty times. This is a calming breathing technique which allows Ki to circulate naturally throughout your body.

MUDRA

Mudra is a Sanskrit word which means "to seal." This word, which has been adopted into Chinese, Korean, and Japanese Ki meditative terminology, describes a hand gesture in which the hand is formed into a specified shape. This shaping of the hand is then used as a meditation tool.

As the fingers are the end points of several of the meridians, Ki naturally flows to them and then away from them. As the Sanskrit meaning of *mudra* implies, when the fingers are formed into a specified pattern, Ki energy is sealed and directed back into the body, instead of being allowed to flow freely out of the fingers and away from the body.

• Ki *Mudra* Meditation •

Assume a kneeling position. If your body does not feel comfortable kneeling, you may sit comfortably in a chair. In either case, your spine must remain erect. See figure 21, pages 88-90.

The *mudra* which is used in connection with Ki meditation is the "Mudra of Body and Mind Unification." This *mudra* is formed by facing both of your palms toward you and then interlocking your fingers. This interlocking process is accomplished by placing the little finger of your

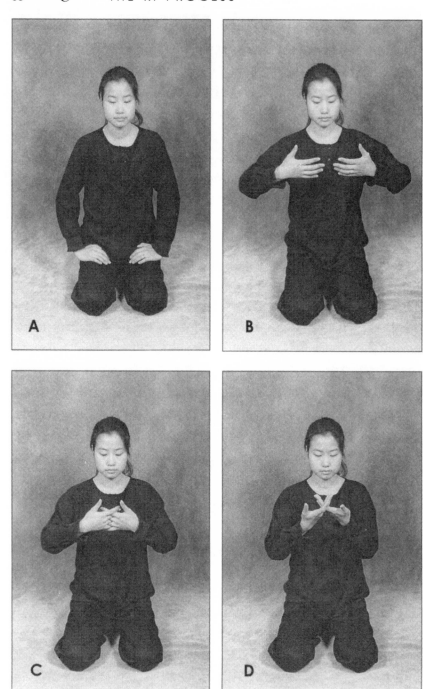

Figure 21. Ki *Mudra* Meditation.

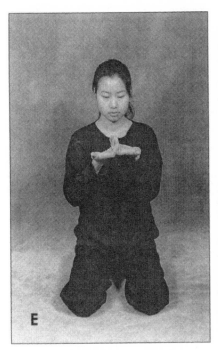
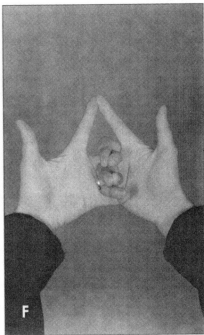

Figure 21 continued.

left hand over the little finger of your right hand, and then allowing the other fingers to continue interlocking in the same pattern. Your forefingers remain pointing naturally outward. Now bend the three interlocked fingers of each hand inward at knuckle level, and toward one another, until the fingertip of each finger is lightly touching its opposing fingertip. With this movement, your forefingers straighten outward and meet. Permit your forefinger tips to meet and point straight upward. Place the thumb of your right hand in between the thumb and forefinger of your left hand. Have your left thumb cross over your right thumb and take its position in a similar location on the right hand. The *mudra* is complete, and your body will begin to experience subtle changes in its circulation of Ki.

Place the *mudra* at eye level, approximately three inches in front of your face. Practice the Four Phase Breath in a natural pattern. Allow your eyes to remain open for a time and study this *mudra* as you breathe. When you feel you have the image of the *mudra* etched in your mind, you

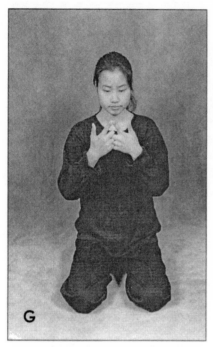

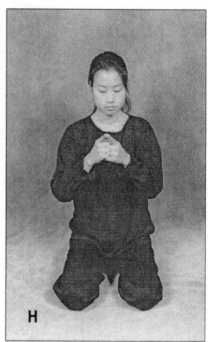

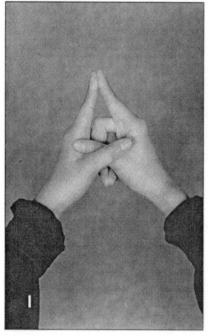

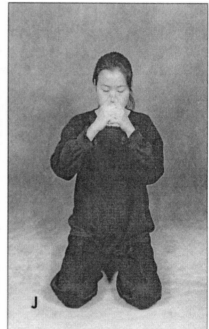

Figure 21 continued.

may close your eyes, while still concentrating on this form. Continue your Four Phase Breath.

It takes practice to develop the ability to maintain the *mudra* held in this upward position for more than a few minutes. If your arms begin to feel tired while keeping the *mudra* intact, allow them to rest on your lap. Your mental image of the *mudra*, however, should remain in its upward-pointing position.

The *Mudra* of Body and Mind Unification is very important for the person who desires to refine his or her Ki. As we have discussed, the average person goes through life with only an unconscious link between body and mind. This *mudra* physically links meridians which affect both elements. Through the use of this *mudra*, your body and mind are given a direct physical method for coming in contact with one another.

This *mudra* meditation may be used initially to link body with mind. As Ki practitioners, through this meditation, become more and more aware of the subtle Ki energy which circulates in the body, they will begin to notice obvious manifestations of their own personal interrelation with life and the universe. In addition, when life problems occur, this is the ideal meditation to put into practice, for through the practice of this body and mind *mudra* meditation, clear insights into problem-solving ideas continually will reveal themselves.

Meditation should not simply be practiced when the mind is ill at ease and you are looking for easy answers. Meditation must be an ongoing practice, used both in times of calm and times of agitation. Meditation is not a drug, though through its practice you can come to a clearer understanding of yourself, the universe, and how you can calmly walk through life.

Use these Ki-oriented meditation exercises to come to a deeper, clearer understanding of how Ki enters, circulates, and emanates from your body. From this, your knowledge and understanding of Ki will continue to grow effortlessly.

KI-DEFINING EXERCISES

Once your breath, body, and mind are consciously focused into one cohesive unit, you can move forward with Ki refinement and begin to perform specific physical Ki-enhancement exercises to facilitate the movement of additional Ki into your body. The following techniques will teach you how to bring your breathing into direct relationship with the physical movements of your body. From this, specific meridians will be stimulated, directing expanded amounts of Ki energy to particular locations in your body.

• Standing *Tan Jun* Breathing Exercise •

Begin by standing with your feet apart (figure 22a), slightly wider than your shoulders. Bend your elbows at a forty-five degree angle and extend your fingers straight ahead in a relaxed fashion. Allow your fingers to be loosely separated. Allow yourself a moment to become comfortable in this position. Visualize your breath entering your body through your nose and extending downward toward your *Tan Jun* (figure 22b).

Now, take in a conscious deep breath through your nose. Observe the air as it enters your body. Direct this breath to your *Tan Jun*. As this breath comes into your body, in a slow natural fashion, allow your knees to bend slightly and your torso to move lower slowly. This kneebend should not be forced. This is not a muscle developing exercise. Allow it to be slow and natural (figure 22c).

In association with your intake of breath and the bending of your knees, extend your arms forward, straight out in front of you. Stretch out your arms slowly, from shoulder level, to the point where your elbows maintain a slight natural bend (figure 22d).

The breathing in and the body movements associated with this Ki exercise should take place simultaneously. Your body begins to move with the beginning of the incoming breath. The physical movement stops once a full breath is taken in.

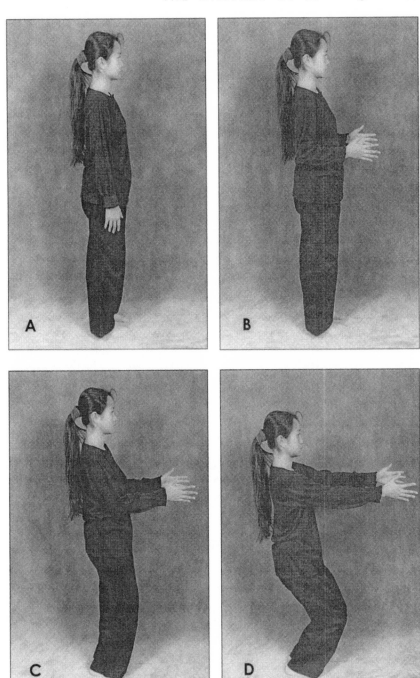

Figure 22. Standing *Tan Jun* Breathing Exercise.

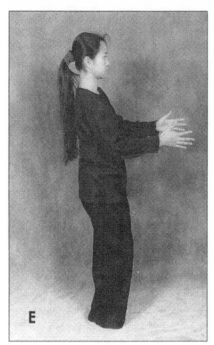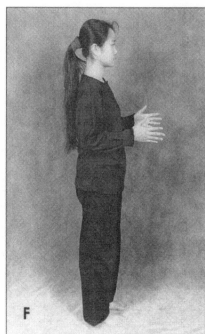

Figure 22 continued.

Once you have reached the completion of your intake of breath, allow this breath to remain casually locked in your *Tan Jun*. Maintain the breath as you hold your arms extended, your fingers outstretched, and your knees and torso in their lowered position (figure 22e). While in this position, allow your body to feel the Ki energy pulsating from your *Tan Jun*, moving up through your body, out along the meridians which reach out through your arms to your hands. Feel how Ki is directed downward to your lower body via the meridians which run the length of your legs to your feet (figure 22f).

Do not hold the breath for an unnatural amount of time. When you feel naturally that it is time to let it out, do so. Watch this breath exit your body from your *Tan Jun*, out through your nose. As the breath leaves you, allow your body to return to the first position of this exercise.

This exercise is not only a *Tan Jun*-focusing technique; it also allows Ki to emanate throughout your body. This Ki generation occurs because virtually all of the meridians are consciously put into motion and stimulated. Thus additional Ki flow is activated throughout your entire body.

DYNAMIC TENSION EXERCISES

Dynamic Tension is a method of tightening the muscles and tendons of a specific bodily region, thus causing additional blood flow to the area. From these exercises, the meridians which are associated with the tensed body parts are highly stimulated. Therefore Ki rushes to them from the *Tan Jun* in a strong directed flow. (See figure 23 on pages 96-97).

Note: Ki-oriented, Dynamic Tension Exercises are a more radical form of Ki enhancement in the human body. Therefore, they should not be performed until the previous developmental techniques in this book have been clearly understood.

• Boulder Push Exercise •

Begin in a standing position, with your hands loosely at your sides. Perform two complete Four Phase Breaths while focalizing your Ki at your *Tan Jun* (figure 23a).

With a new intake of breath through your nose, move your left leg forward, as if you were about to take a step. As the breath comes in and the step is taken, bend your elbows slightly and turn your wrists until your open palms are facing upward, at approximately your waist level (figure 23b).

Once your intake of breath is complete, allow the breath to remain locked in your *Tan Jun*. Feel the Ki energy radiate as you bring your upward-facing palms along the side of your body to chest level. Once at chest level, allow your open palms to turn outward and face in front of you (figure 23c and d).

As you exhale your breath, tighten all the muscles of your shoulders, back, arms, and hands. Powerfully push forward with your open palms, visualizing a large boulder in front of you which moves with the

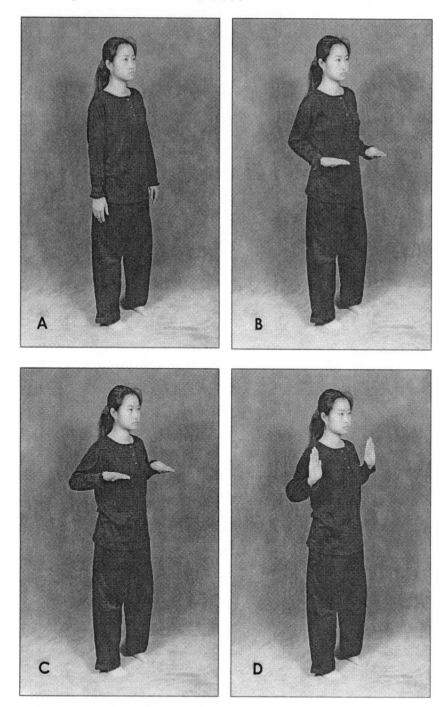

Figure 23. Boulder Push Exercise.

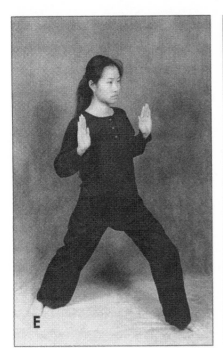

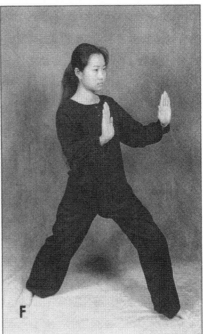

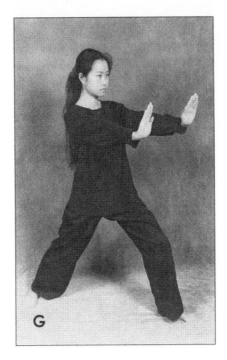

Figure 23 continued.

power of your push. As your arms extend, allow your left arm to remain slightly in front, your right arm slightly behind, pushing forward (figure 23e, f, and g). Once your breath is exhaled completely, observe the emptiness for a moment as your arms remain extended, feeling the Ki radiating from them.

When the time comes to take a new breath, breathe in, gracefully returning to your original standing position with your hands loosely at your sides. When the breath is complete, feel how full of Ki your arms and hands have become. Allow the breath to exit naturally, feeling the Ki remaining.

As you begin your next breath, step forward with your right leg and perform the same exercise on your right side.

The Boulder Push Exercise is ideal for focalizing Ki into your arms, shoulders, and hands when you are anticipating the need to perform strenuous physical movements with them. This is because this exercise stimulates the meridians of these limbs, thus providing additional Ki power to them.

• Upper Body Ki Exercise •

In a standing position, separate your legs until they are approximately four inches beyond shoulder width (figure 24a). Once you have obtained this stance, lower your upper torso by bending your knees slightly. In this position, your body becomes very secure. Straighten your spine (figure 24b). Extend your arms up over your head, allowing them to meet and cross at wrist level. Your fingers are extended upward (figure 24c)

Take an initial deep breath. Send it to your *Tan Jun* and hold it for a moment. Feel how your *Tan Jun* is stimulated with Ki. Release your breath.

Breathe in deeply as you tighten the muscles of your arms, chest, back, and shoulders. Direct your arms (still crossed at wrist level), slowly yet powerfully down in front of you, until they are perpendicular to the ground. Feel them vibrate from the power. Hold this breath and position for a moment (figure 24d).

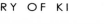

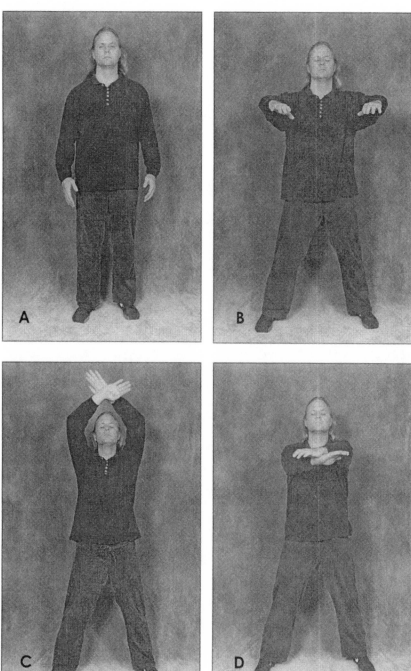

Figure 24. Upper Body Ki Exercise.

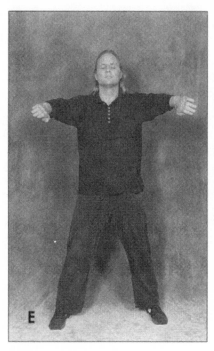 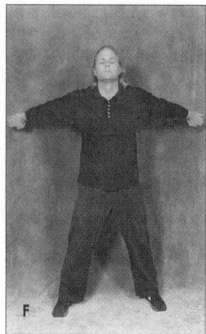

Figure 24 continued.

Release the breath. As you do so, powerfully send your straightened arms back to shoulder level, hands open, as if you were swimming. Stop your arms when they become even with your body (figure 24e, f).

Allow yourself to remain empty of air for a natural amount of time, witnessing the Ki permeating the space in front of you and exiting through your chest. When you feel it is time, return to the first position and repeat this exercise five times.

From this exercise, the meridians which inhabit your arms, chest, back, and, to a lesser degree, your legs are substantially stimulated, thereby creating added Ki intake and transport. As your arms are sent outward, the Ki of this exercise is focused on your chest. This is a very beneficial exercise to practice before you must encounter people or situations you know mean you no good. When people unconsciously sense that powerful Ki energy is emanating from you, they do not attempt to cause you harm.

• Ki Leg Exercise •

From a standing position, open your legs and consciously place them approximately four inches beyond shoulder width. Bend your knees slightly, assuming a firm stance (figure 25a and b).

Once your legs are firmly located and you feel comfortable with your stance, perform a few natural Four Phase Breaths. As you do, begin to visualize Ki entering the bottom of your feet from the ground as you breathe in. With each intake breath, see golden Ki enter your feet, illuminating your *Tan Jun*, and permeating your body. As your breath goes out, feel yourself becoming more and more grounded in your thoughts and physical actions. With additional breaths, feel the essence of Mother Earth coming in and nourishing your being.

Once you feel you have anchored yourself successfully to the Earth, allow your hands to rise up to waist level, gently bending your elbows.

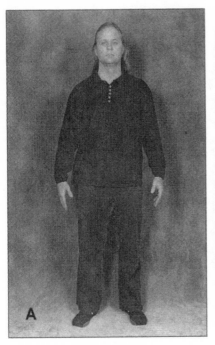
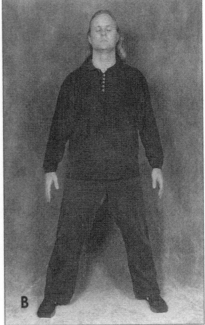

Figure 25. Ki Leg Exercise.

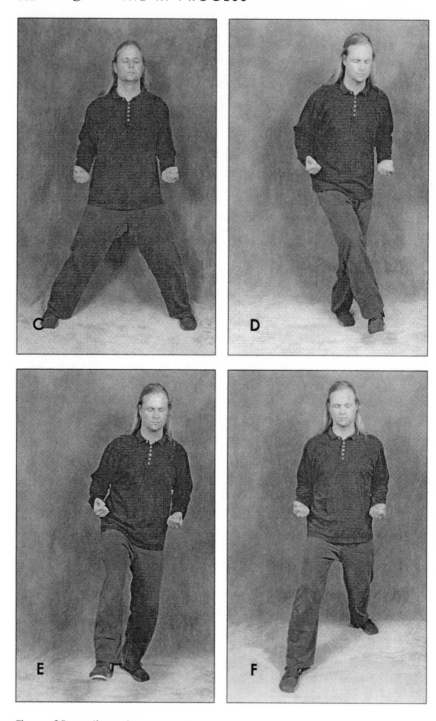

Figure 25 continued.

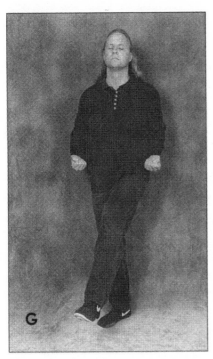 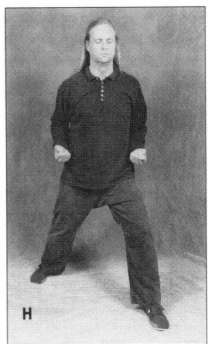

Figure 25 continued.

Once your hands reach this position, form them into fists. While making these fists, do not force your fingers into your palms. Instead, allow them to be naturally closed, sealing Ki energy within them (figure 25c).

Once you have achieved this position, begin your conscious intake of breath. As you do, lift your right leg approximately two inches from the ground (figure 25d). Swing it, in a circular fashion, out in front of your left leg. Tighten the upper muscles of the leg just enough so that there is a very conscious awareness of their involvement in this movement. Then allow the leg to swing forward, as if stepping, landing approximately two feet from where its movement began. Once at rest, straighten your left leg naturally as you bend your right knee. Then exhale (figure 25e, f).

As this leg motion is in progress, feel the grounding balance your left leg maintains as your right leg is in motion. Once the right leg has again touched the Earth, feel the enormous amount of Ki energy which enters your body as a result of the movement.

With your next breath, direct your left leg in a circular pattern as before, in front of your right leg. When the stepping movement has been completed, consciously allow your left foot to impact Mother Earth and embrace her Ki energy (figure 25g, h).

If space permits, move forward approximately four steps in this circular walking motion. If desired, you can consciously turn your body and perform this exercise again in the opposite direction.

This exercise stimulates the meridians which extend along the legs and culminate in your feet. It promotes an added sense of balance, and also provides the awakened practitioner with a conscious sense of the Ki energy of the Earth flowing into the body through the feet.

• Kneeling Ki-Empowerment Exercise •

Assume a kneeling position (figure 26, pages 105-106). Place your hands naturally on your lap. Close your eyes and begin to perform the Four Phase Breath naturally for a few minutes, centering yourself (figure 26a).

When your mind has been calmed from external stimuli, place your hands to the sides of your waist. Your palms should be open and facing upward. Tense the muscles and tendons of your fingers, forming what is known as a knife hand (figure 26b).

When you feel you are ready, take a deep breath in through your nose, sending it to your *Tan Jun*. As this breath is coming in, extend your arms upward in front of your body with all of the strength of your arms, back, and shoulders, until your two open palms reach a pinnacle just above your head (figure 26c and d).

At this point, your intake of breath should be complete. Feel how the Ki energy of the Earth has entered into your body, in association with the Ki energy of the air coming to you through your breath. Breathe out, as your hands return to their position at your sides (figure 26 e, f, g).

This exercise is ideal for developing added overall Ki circulation and strength when the need for them is immanent. This exercise should not be implemented more than three times in any given week by the Ki novice,

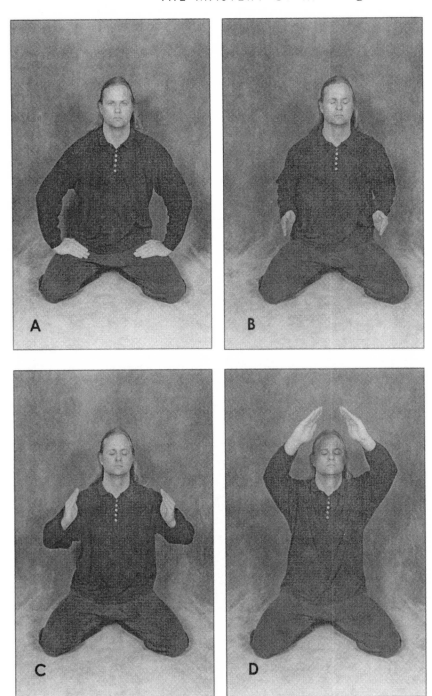

Figure 26. Kneeling Ki-Empowerment Exercise.

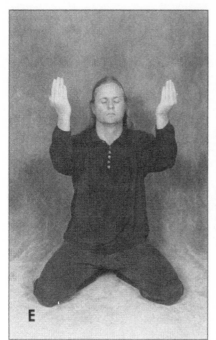

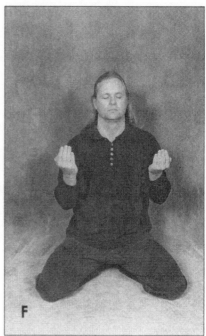

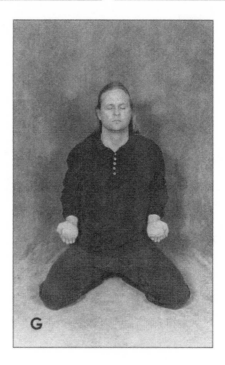

Figure 26 continued.

however. In addition, the actual physical repetition of this exercise should not be performed more than three times in any given session, since it forces excessive amounts of Ki into the body. Excessive amounts of Ki can substantially elevate blood pressure, or can be overwhelming to those Ki practitioners not adequately prepared to consciously direct the overabundance of Ki energy into the physical or mental element actually desired.

Through observation of ethereal body mechanics and practice of Ki exercises, the Ki enthusiast will come effortlessly to understand how to direct Ki consciously where it is most needed in the body or mind. As in all Ki practices, Ki should never be forced; it should simply be allowed to enter, pass through the body, and then leave as nature intended.

• Ki Hand-Focalizing Exercise •

As we learned from the meridian study and from the Mudra Meditation Exercise, the hands are the bodily location where several meridians culminate. Thus Ki naturally flows to the fingertips. In order to utilize the Ki which emanates from the hands effectively, you must consciously learn to draw it out. (See figure 27, pages 108-110.)

Stand with your legs apart, at slightly more than shoulder width. Allow your knees to bend slightly. Place your hands in front of you and vigorously rub them together for approximately thirty seconds, or until you feel heat emanating from them (figure 27a and b).

Stand with your spine erect and place your hands in front of your torso, bending both of your elbows at a forty-five degree angle. Have your left hand facing upward and your right hand facing downward, one directly above the other and approximately one inch from one another. Feel the heat exchange between your two hands (figure 27c).

Take an initial deep breath. Direct it to your *Tan Jun*. Hold it for a moment and feel the Ki pulsating throughout your body. Allow the breath to flow out of you and embrace the emptiness. Close your eyes. Begin to practice a natural Four Phase Breath.

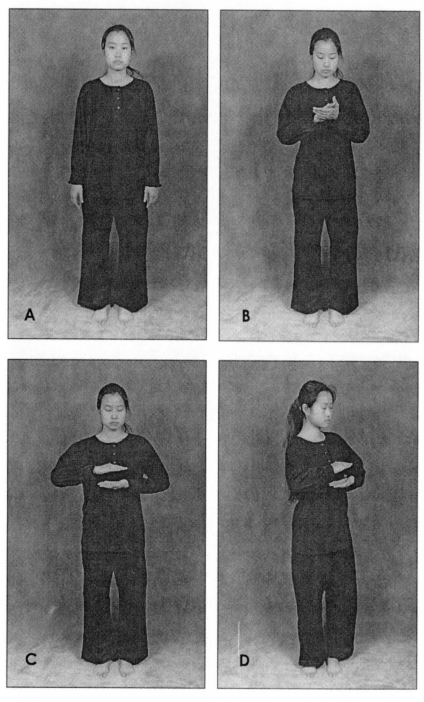

Figure 27. Ki Hand-Focalizing Exercise.

While leaving your hands in place, gently pivot your upper torso from the base of your spine, first to the left side and then to the right. Pivoting in this slow, controlled manner stimulates the meridians which run along your spine (figure 27d, e, f).

Perform this pivoting motion three times. As you come to the fourth pivot, separate your hands. Have your right hand travel in the direction of your left elbow and your left hand slowly move toward your right elbow. As you pivot back the fifth time, allow your elbows to move outward, so your hands will pass over one another. Feel the Ki exchanging between your two hands, as one moves over the other.

As soon as your pivot is complete, flip your hands over so the right hand is facing up and the left hand is facing down. As you pivot back this time, again allow your hands to move slowly past one another, exchanging Ki. With each pivot, allow your hands to change position as they move past one another exchanging Ki (figure 27 g, h, and i).

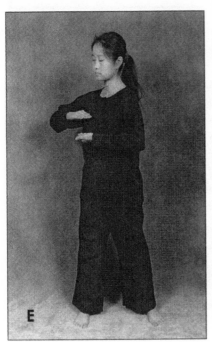
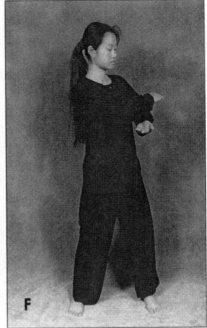

Figure 27 continued.

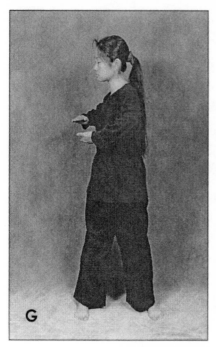

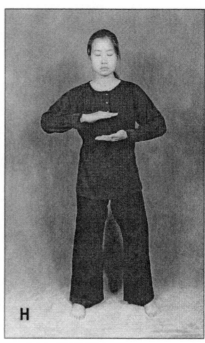

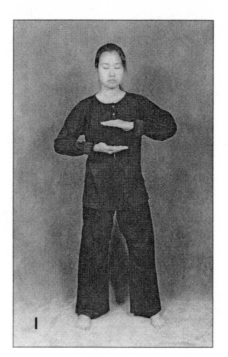

Figure 27 continued.

Perform this exercise for approximately five minutes. The Ki energy which has developed in your hands will become quite noticeable. You can use this Ki energy to aid in acupressure massage or other necessary tasks.

EXTENDING YOUR KI

Ki is a consciousness. Those who understand the existence of Ki have the ability to learn how to focus this very powerful energy consciously and direct it outside the body. Those who have no knowledge of Ki remain unaware and are controlled by the random energies of the world around them.

To extend Ki energy, you must first possess an adequate amount of it. If you attempt to extend your Ki and have not developed the proper channeling methods (as described in this book), your results will be minimal and you will leave yourself completely robbed of all energy. Therefore, to extend your Ki, you must first achieve a very refined state of mind.

If you have developed the necessary Ki-channeling knowledge, you know that the extension of Ki cannot be forced like the lifting of a heavy weight. The extension of Ki energy is simply a method of allowing Ki to enter the body naturally, gather in the *Tan Jun*, and then be directed outward in a natural manner.

• Ki-Extension Exercise •

From a standing position, focus your attention and consciously begin to perform The Four Phase Breath. Once you feel calm, with your breath centered in your *Tan Jun*, extend one of your arms naturally out to one side. Allow your elbow to remain bent, so your arm does not become strained. Leave your hand open, with your fingers loosely outstretched. Once your body has achieved a comfortable balanced state in this position, begin to visualize Ki energy entering in the form of golden light with each intake of breath; feel it congregating in your *Tan Jun*. As you exhale,

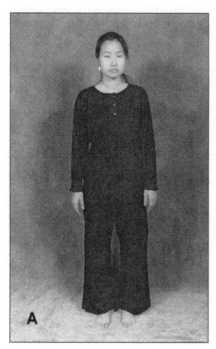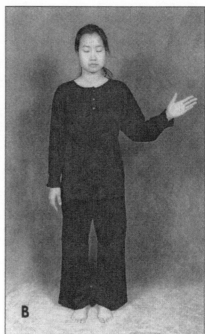

Figure 28. Ki-Extension Exercise.

visualize this Ki extending up your body, out your arm, and exiting through your fingers (see figure 28).

As you practice this exercise, witness how first your upper arm, then your lower arm, and finally your hand and fingers begin to feel more and more strength with each exhalation, as Ki travels from your *Tan Jun* out to your fingers. Experience the strength your hand feels as Ki energy emanates from your fingers.

Soundwaves cannot be seen, yet they are experienced. When practicing this exercise, allow the Ki to flow outward from your fingers as a sound speaker disperses music to the environment around it. Mentally observe the Ki energy flowing from your fingers as it dissipates into the atmosphere surrounding you.

As you begin to feel the Ki power and energy which you have consciously directed from your hand with this Ki-Extension Exercise, lower your arm and begin to focus and then extend this same Ki energy from any part of your body. Simply focus your mind, concentrate on your *Tan Jun*, breathe your Ki energy in, and then witness it extending from any precise location of the body you desire.

KI INFUSION

As we have learned in the various Ki understandings and techniques described in this book, the hands and the feet are great resources for the channeling of Ki, as they are the endpoints of various meridians. Once you consciously bring Ki into your body, you can disperse it easily through the touching of your hands, whenever an individual is in need of your help in their healing. To accomplish this Ki infusion into the body of another person readily, first perform the previous Ki-Extension Exercise and then apply appropriate touch therapy to the prescribed *Hyel* on the body which accesses the meridian with a blockage of Ki. In this way, you will not only provide suitable healing stimulation to the *Hyel,* you can also greatly aid in the rapid overall healing process, as Ki is being consciously infused into the patient's body.

This conscious extension of Ki, emanating from the hands or the feet, is the same practice which advanced martial artists put to use when they deliver powerful punching or kicking techniques. As you come to master Ki through continued experiential understanding and practice, you will be able to direct it from any element of your body with simply the slightest of thoughts.

KI EMANATION

Ki emanation around your entire body in times of physical or psychic peril can be accomplished effectively by performing a slight variation of the Ki-Extension Exercise previously detailed. In the case of full-body Ki emanation, first consciously bring excess amounts of Ki into your body via your breath and direct it toward your *Tan Jun*. Begin to visualize Ki extending from your *Tan Jun* and encompassing your entire body in a golden bubble.

To become accomplished at full-body Ki emanation, practice this technique in various life situations: when you are standing, sitting, walking, or running. By experiencing the fact that Ki will enter your body readily whenever you successfully open yourself to it, and by experiencing your ability to direct Ki outward from your being at will, you will come to know that Ki emanation is not something abstract or unobtainable. In times of true need, you can successfully access Ki at will.

It is important to remember that Ki is a mental understanding. It is not a physical manifestation such as the growth of a muscle when a weight is lifted. Ki is a mental science. Just as positive thoughts have been proven to possess a beneficial effect over all aspects of your physical and mental being, Ki energy derives its strength from this same positive mental acceptance of your mind.

PHYSICAL STRENGTH VERSUS KI

Physical strength is not limitless strength. Physical strength, such as heightened muscle development, is a process of body enhancement which is achieved easily by prescribed physical weightlifting exercises. This type of strength development, however, is quickly lost when the exercises are discontinued. Muscle development is, therefore, a temporary form of strength. When you develop internal strength through the use of Ki, on the other hand, you never lose your understanding of how to access Ki effectively. This form of internal strength and energy is always available to you.

KI IN DAILY LIFE

Ki is not a vain energy for use by the power hungry or people defined by negative emotions and selfish desires. These mindsets are self-destructive and lead one to a life with a complete lack of peace. If such people attempt to focalize Ki energy toward negative ends, their own self-defeatist emotions hinder them from developing the proper channels through which the positive, life-giving energy of Ki can pass. Ki energy is, however, readily available and usable to those with the right frame of mind.

Those who make positive Ki-development exercises a part of their daily lives already emanate large amounts of Ki. When you come into contact with them, this positive life-giving energy is obvious. These are people who always attract positive events in their lives; negative occurrences do not seek them out. Why? Because Ki is a positive energy and, therefore, it strikes a sympathetic chord with other positive energies, events, and people of this universe.

When it comes time for Ki-refined individuals to focalize their Ki energy and deliver it as an aid in healing or as a method to send positive energy to others, they willingly open themselves up to the degree where added Ki naturally passes through them and they are more than willing to extend it to those around them.

KI AND THE ENVIRONMENT

Have you ever entered into a new environment and immediately felt very peaceful? Or the reverse: have you ever gone into a place and immediately felt ill at ease? As you now understand, the universe is filled with energy. This energy can be taken in and used by everyone. If you take in this energy and put it to very positive use, you fill your surroundings with positive Ki energy. The same is true if you are very negative. You take in energy and dispense it negatively. In this world, good is always good and bad is always bad. Strive to embrace the universal Ki energy in positive ways.

There are times when you will encounter situations in your life where you do not feel comfortable because you feel the negative energy left in a place by previous occupants. When you come into contact with negative environments that you must endure, the solution is to cleanse the energy of the area with positive Ki energy.

There are two ways you can fill a negative environment with positive energy. The first is to open the structure up to new, clean air as much as possible. Open the windows. Open the doors. As universal Ki is continually in circulation and is based in a positive creative source, this influx of new energy quickly cleanses the surroundings. This is also the best method for dealing with a very negative person with whom you must remain in close proximity on an ongoing basis.

If there is no way to effectively open the structure to fresh air, then you must first become very aware of the source of the negative energy surrounding you. By understanding that it is something external to yourself, you will prevent yourself from being overtaken or controlled by it and will thus already have freed yourself from its negative impact. The main thing to remember is that you cannot control the emotions or energies of another person; you can only control your own. With this knowledge in mind, do not set out to immediately and forcefully alter the negative energy left in a specific environment by another person or persons. Instead, focus your Ki energy on whatever task is at hand, remaining positive, and the environment around you will change, naturally and gradually, to one permeated with positive Ki energy.

THE QUICK FIX KI STIMULATION GUIDE

In times of physical or emotional distress it is important to remember that you, as a conscious Ki practitioner, now possess the refined ability to rapidly tap into the boundless universal energy known as Ki. From this, you can reenergize your physical strength when you are too weak to take another step, or you can receive clear mental perceptions when you are too emotionally drained to think another thought.

Under adverse conditions the mind often does not wish to embrace the fact that you can take control over any life situation and shift its balance in your favor. As a Ki practitioner, under any condition, you must remind yourself that you can consciously draw in Ki energy to aid you in your times of need; all that is required is that you focus your mental intent and consciously allow Ki to enter your body.

As you now understand, from following the practices outlined in this book, your Ki energy is directly related to your breath. Therefore, the easiest and most effective way for you to draw a large amount of Ki energy into your body, in times of need, is through conscious breathing.

The most effective technique to use to instantly revitalize your body and mind is the Four Phase Breath Exercise (previously described, page 77 ff.). Whenever you need reaffirmation that Ki energy is constantly available to you, close your eyes and breathe that life-giving Ki energy into your body; watch it enter through your nose in a golden flow of light and congregate in your *Tan Jun*. Once your in-breath is complete, hold

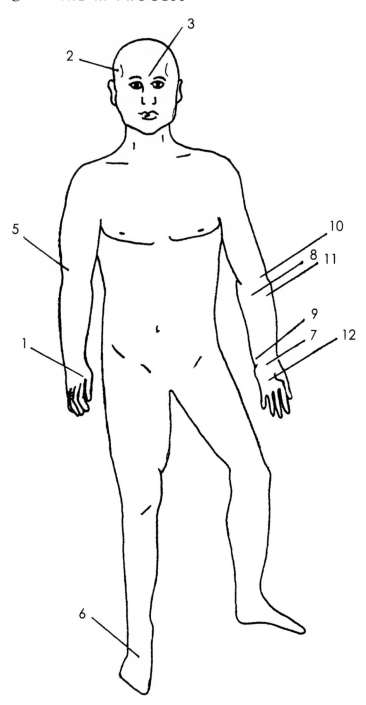

Figure 29. *Hyel* points.

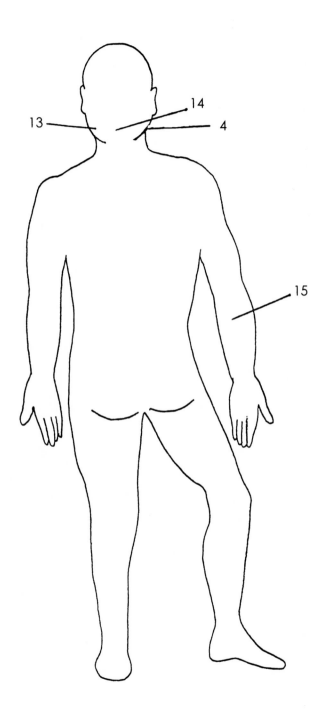

Figure 29 continued.

that golden breath in place for a moment and embrace its power. As you release it, let go of all negativity, weakness, and confusion. You will be revitalized and your Ki force will be stimulated.

ACUPRESSURE QUICK FIXES

At times in life we all encounter periods when a particular function of our bodies is not performing properly, or we are suffering from symptoms, such as a headache or nausea, brought about by external stimuli. In these times, there are *Hyel*, which when stimulated properly, promise, at least, temporary relief from these conditions. See figure 29 (pages 118-119) which illustrates the pressure points. These pressure points, when stimulated properly with the information provided, will help you relieve some of the very common adverse physical and mental conditions you may find yourself suffering from.

Headache

Hyel Number 1: This *Hyel* is ideally suited to aid in the remedy of frontal headaches.

Take your thumb and apply firm pressure. Allow this pressure to remain constant for approximately one minute. Remove your thumb from this *Hyel* for thirty seconds, then again apply pressure for thirty seconds. Again, remove the thumb for thirty seconds and then replace it for an additional thirty seconds of firm pressure.

Hyel Number 2: Stimulating of this *Hyel* is effective in aiding in the recovery from side and rear headaches.

With both your left and your right forefinger, apply pressure to these *Hyel* on both sides of your head. Do not massage, as is the common reaction. Instead, hold firm pressure for forty-five seconds and then release.

Wait for three minutes and then perform this *Hyel*-stimulating technique again for forty-five seconds more.

Hyel Number 3: This *Hyel* activates Ki, which aids in the recovery from sinus headaches.

Close your eyes. Take the middle finger of your right hand and apply firm pressure for two minutes. Take your finger away and remain at rest, with your eyes closed, for two minutes. Take the middle finger of your left hand and apply pressure to this *Hyel*. Allow the pressure to remain for two minutes.

Indigestion

Hyel Numbers 4 and 5: Lean your head slightly forward and close your eyes. Place the middle finger of your right hand at *Hyel Number 4* on the right side of your skull. Hold it firmly in position for two minutes. Remove it. Take your left thumb and apply pressure to *Hyel Number 5*, located on your right arm. Allow pressure to remain on this *Hyel* for two minutes. Remove your thumb from this acupressure location, and rest for one minute. Perform the same pressure point stimulation on the opposite side of your body, using the middle finger of your left hand on the left side of your skull, and the thumb of your right hand on your left arm for the same two minute intervals.

Constipation

Hyel Number 6: Locate the *Hyel* on the top of both your feet. Take the middle finger of both the right and left hand, and place firm pressure on these *Hyel*. Hold for one minute and then release. Wait for two minutes and then apply pressure again for one minute. Release, wait one minute, and then apply appropriate pressure one final time for one minute.

Chest Pain

Hyel Number 7: Take the first finger of your left hand and place it on this *Hyel*, which is located on your right wrist. Close your eyes and consciously breathe slowly. Hold this pressure point for three minutes.

PMS

Hyel Number 8: Close your eyes. Take a deep breath and release it. Take your left thumb and apply pressure to this *Hyel*, on your right arm, for one minute. Remove your pressure. Relax for one minute. Take a second deep breath and release. Take your right thumb and apply pressure to this *Hyel*, on your left arm, for one minute. Release and relax.

Menstrual Cramps

Hyel Number 9: Located on the inside of your upper wrist. Apply pressure with your right middle finger for three minutes.

Male Sexual Functions

Hyel Numbers 10 and 11: These two *Hyel* work together. Therefore they should be stimulated simultaneously with your first and middle finger. Locate these *Hyel* (on either side of your inner elbow crease) and apply pressure for one minute. Release and apply pressure for two minutes. These *Hyel* are active on both sides of the body, thus the side which is most comfortable to you can be readily accessed.

Anxiety

Hyel Number 12: Close your eyes. Take several very slow, very conscious deep breaths. Open your left palm; face it upward. Take the first finger of your right hand and apply pressure to this *Hyel*, located in your central palm, for two minutes, as you consciously observe your breath entering your body through your nose and progressing to your *Tan Jun*. Release the pressure. Open the palm of your right palm. Take the first finger of your left hand and locate this *Hyel*. Again hold it for two minutes as you consciously observe the Ki breath entering your body.

Fatigue or Weakness

Hyel Number 13: Locate this *Hyel* with the first finger of your left hand, and apply pressure to the rear right side of your skull, two inches behind your ear. Apply pressure for two minutes. As you do, consciously bring added breath into your body through your nose by consciously breathing in approximately twice your normal resting intake of air. Focus the energy of your breath in your *Tan Jun*. Release pressure from the *Hyel* and return to normal breathing. Wait three minutes and repeat the process one more time.

Lightheadedness

Hyel Number 14: Close your eyes. Take three slow deep breaths. With your left middle finger locate this *Hyel* at the top of your spine and apply pressure to it for three minutes. As you do, remain very concentrated on your breath. Consciously guide your breath in and out of your nose, accessing the Ki energy in your *Tan Jun*.

Insomnia

Hyel Number 15: Insomnia is greatly relieved by performing the Kneeling Abdominal Breathing Meditation Exercise previously detailed in this text (page 85). Perform this breathing exercise for approximately five minutes. Upon completion of this breath practice, lie down for sleep. Access the *Hyel* on the outer section of your left forearm with your right forefinger. Allow any thoughts which enter your mind to be like ocean waves, coming in and then naturally leaving. Do not attempt to control them. Hold this *Hyel* for five minutes, and as your mind rests, you will sleep.

It is important to remember that the lifestyle you choose to live will directly affect how your body reacts to the various elements it comes into contact with. Thus, acupressure should not be approached as a cure-all to conditions which can be more consciously relieved with a proper diet, exercise, the right mental attitude, and meditation. Additionally, many symptoms, such as neck pain and lower back pain, are more a condition of fatigued muscles than inadequate Ki flow along a specific meridian pathway. Therefore, massage will be more advantageous to aid in the relief of these conditions than will acupressure.

CONCLUSION

You have now come to understand that the refinement of Ki takes place through conscious effort. From the continued practice of the Ki-focalizing techniques outlined in this book, you can rapidly develop a comprehensive, interactive understanding of Ki. As you progress along the path of unending Ki knowledge, no longer will Ki be some abstract power. It will be a prevalent, unlimited, and useable source of energy in all aspects of your everyday life.

Ki energy is universally available. Feel the Ki.

INDEX

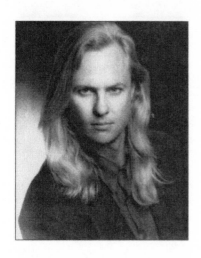

ABOUT THE AUTHOR

Scott Shaw is a martial arts instructor, actor, and filmmaker. He began studying the martial arts as a young boy and at 21 was a certified Master Instructor in the Korean Martial Arts of Hapkido and Taekwondo. He was certified 7th Degree Black Belt Master by the Korean Hapkido Federation, making him one of the most advanced non-Korean Masters of the art of Hapkido in the world. Shaw has been a prolific writer, with articles appearing in magazines such as *Inside Karate, Black Belt, Martial Art Movies, Secrets of the Masters,* and *Inside Taekwondo.* He is co-editor of *The Tuttle Dictionary of the Martial Arts of Korea, China & Japan* (Tuttle 1996), *Hapkido: The Korean Art of Self-Defense* (Tuttle 1997), and is a contributor to the *Martial Arts Source Book* (HarperCollins 1994).

CPSIA information can be obtained
at www.ICGtesting.com
Printed in the USA
FSOW01n1248180416
19372FS